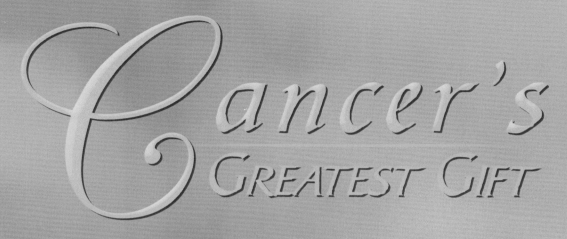

Cancer's
GREATEST GIFT

Keys to Radiant Health and Joy

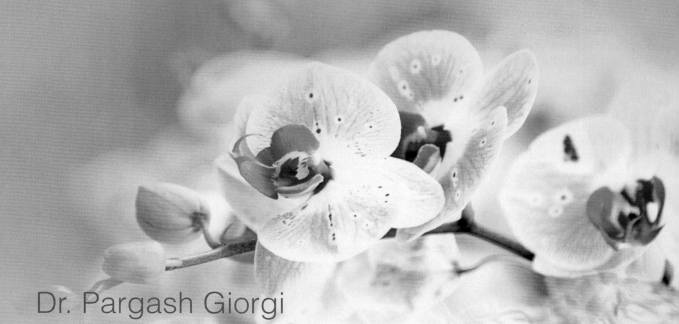

Dr. Pargash Giorgi

To order additional copies of this book, contact:
Xlibris
1-888-795-4274
www.Xlibris.com
Orders@Xlibris.com

ISBN: Softcover   978-1-4771-1649-4
             Hardcover   978-1-4771-1650-0
             E-book   978-1-4771-1651-7

Library of Congress Control Number: 2012909228

Print information available on the last page.

Rev. date: 12/15/2020

DISCLAIMER

Pargash Giorgi is a doctor of philosophy -- not a medical doctor. The advice she offers in this book is not a treatment or cure for any medical condition. You are responsible for its use, misuse, or non-use, just as you are responsible for your own physical, mental, and emotional well-being.

From my perspective as a typically skeptical, western-trained medical doctor, the fact that Pargash has survived and overcome a life-threatening, supposedly "incurable," disease is the ultimate proof that everything she is recommending to others is vital and imperative to follow as a life's prescription.

Because of this, the message is universal, and her words carry an obvious power behind them that needs to be read by everyone . . . . We can all live inspired lives by following her practical, real, down-to-earth yet spiritually based prescriptive advice.

Dr. Arthur Brownstein, M.D., M.P.H., F.A.C.P

Your Free Gift valued at $585

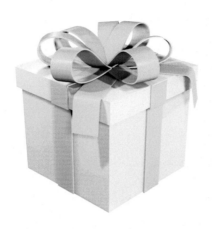

Please visit my website at

Newlifeafterbreastcancer.com

to claim your free gift

Contents

Chapter 6

Chapter 7

APPENDIX A

APPENDIX B

APPENDIX C

APPENDIX D

Foreword

The author of this intriguing book speaks to fellow women who live in fear of cancer or are confused after diagnosis and treatment. Hers are not just kind words of support; readers are strongly invited to change their own life, although for some of them it may be an operation more painful than surgery itself. But the rewards are worthwhile: discover who you are and place your mind in control of your body by overcoming myths and an exaggerated dependency on conventional medicine. Successful followers of this approach may eventually see what initially was a frightening diagnosis of cancer as actually a gift of life. The process of preventing recurrence, enhancing healing, acquiring new personal skills, and improving social and physical life will make them not merely survivors but better people and happier human beings.

Many decades of teaching biomedical sciences have made me aware of the shortcomings of conventional medical approaches: too little prevention and too much treatment of symptoms, within a merely physical view of patients. Enlightened medical texts speak of a new psychosocial medicine; but in practice, a very large proportion of common diseases would be preventable if a healthy lifestyle was adopted (the socio-political aspect) and heavy pharmaceutical treatments would be avoided if a patient-centered medicine was adopted (the psychological aspect). The author takes advantage of such progressive views when advising about overcoming cancer. Her knowledge derives from critical readings, but mostly from personal experience as a breast-cancer patient.

The most interesting aspect of this manual concerns the importance given to resources obtained from the psychological control of our body. Even health-generating nutritional changes ultimately derive from this domain of positive medical psychology. Two operational strategies can be identified: the well-known negative effect of stress and fear on the self-healing capacity of the body and the lesser-known mind power (general attitude and positive declaration) on body functions. One additional psychological tool stressed by the author is becoming aware of the social models that prevent women, since infancy, from being in charge of themselves and making their own decisions. Deciding to adopt alternative (integrative, complementary) medical help is the obvious advantage of such a courageous step, which was also taken by the author during her experience with breast cancer.

Cancer's Greatest Gift is not a book advising breast cancer patients only, but it stands out for its understandable, essential, and rich content, dismissing myths, releasing fears, and opening up to alternative ideas for healing. I would also advise healthy women to read it to unveil the gift of life transformation that would prevent those diseases precipitated by a pathogenic lifestyle.

Dr. Piero Giorgi
Former Senior Lecturer in Biomedical Sciences
University of Queensland, Brisbane

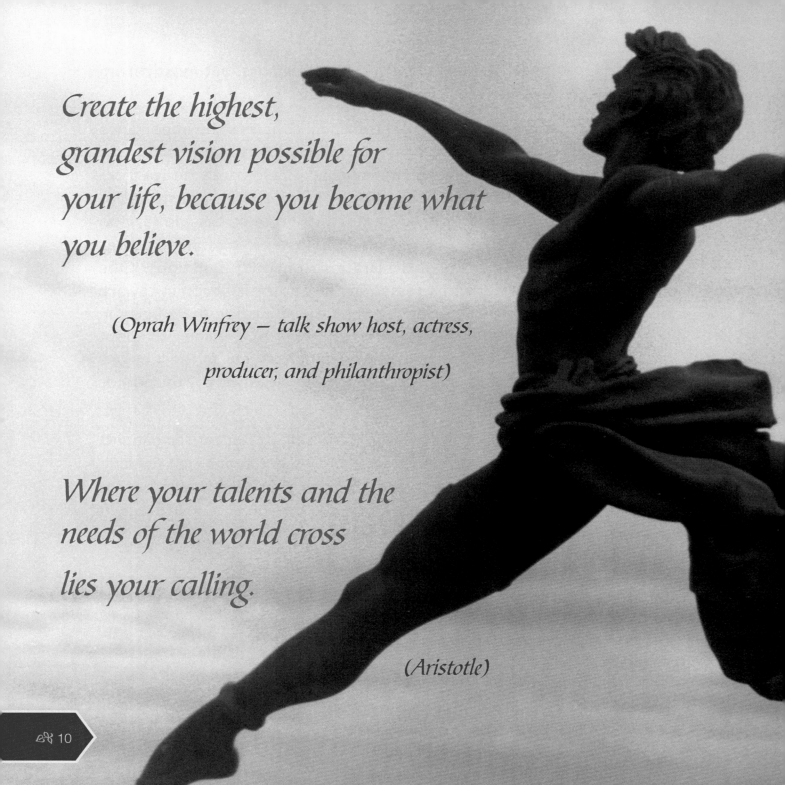

Create the highest,
grandest vision possible for
your life, because you become what
you believe.

(Oprah Winfrey — talk show host, actress, producer, and philanthropist)

Where your talents and the
needs of the world cross
lies your calling.

(Aristotle)

Author's Note

Dear fellow breast cancer recoverer,

This book on breast cancer is written for you. My aim is that once you have read this book, you will not even think about dis-ease or cancer anymore but focus only on how to attain optimal health and beauty beyond belief, regardless of your age. More specifically, in this book I will explain that while there is an understandable tendency for doctors to frown upon self-healing, and I am conscious of the fact that recovery can be delayed if you do not pursue the right path, self-healing has been proven to be extremely effective. From my own experience, I know that there is a place for such a model of recovery if done with the right tools; I have created and used them successfully and so have thousands of other women who have had a history of breast cancer.

Why Read This book?

It is my desire that this book will help you live a life that is:

- happier and free of fear;

- healthier and free of pain;

- worth living and blessed with longevity;

- one in which you will feel good and look great;

- one in which you will easily keep your brain young and sharp;

- one in which you will maintain your perfect weight.

I have gone through many challenges in my life, and it is my deepest joy to share with you the most effective tools and techniques to move from where you are now to the life you've always wanted.

This Book Is for You *If*:

- you've had breast cancer and are worried you may relapse
- you want to get your life back together
- you want to enjoy radiant health
- you want to discover cutting-edge tools and techniques that will enable you to make deep inner change that is permanent;
- you have the willingness and desire to make a commitment to yourself to change your world.

This Book is NOT for You *if*:

- you have no interest in discovering the deeper reason why you developed cancer;
- you don't want to change on a deep level;
- you do not wish to explore new possibilities;
- you want your life to go back to the way it was rather than move forward to something even better.

Life is not about waiting for the storms to pass. It's about learning to dance in the rain.

(Vivian Greene – artist, author, visionary, entrepreneur)

Appreciations

To all my mentors: Thank you for seeing and embracing my uniqueness and guiding me through the production of this book. I immensely appreciate your assistance and reassurance every step of the way.

To Dr. Piero Giorgi: I am grateful to you for offering to write the Foreword in spite of your hectic schedule.

To my friends – Paula Corriea, Hilary Cox, Mark Thornton, Alan Morison, and Kirsten Campbell: a big thank you for providing feedback on various aspects of the book.

And to all my clients: Thank you for giving me the opportunity to help you and to learn ways in which I can help you even more.

I also appreciate all my readers, and I would love your feedback on this book. If you have any questions or comments, please visit this website, where all your questions will be answered:

I would love your feedback on this book, so if you have any questions or comments please go to:

newlifeafterbreastcancer.com

where *all* your questions will be addressed.

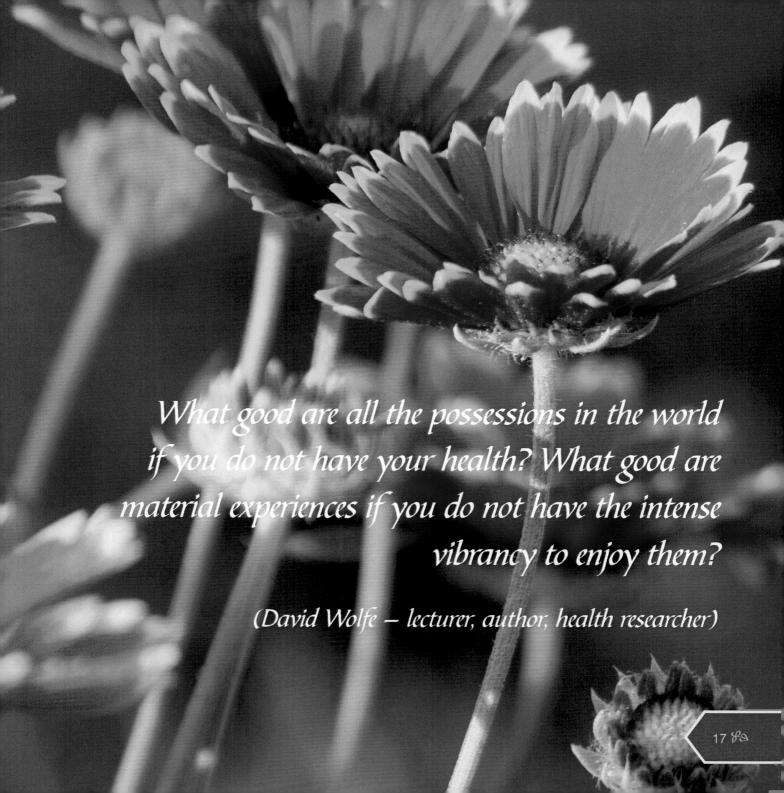

What good are all the possessions in the world if you do not have your health? What good are material experiences if you do not have the intense vibrancy to enjoy them?

(David Wolfe – lecturer, author, health researcher)

Introduction

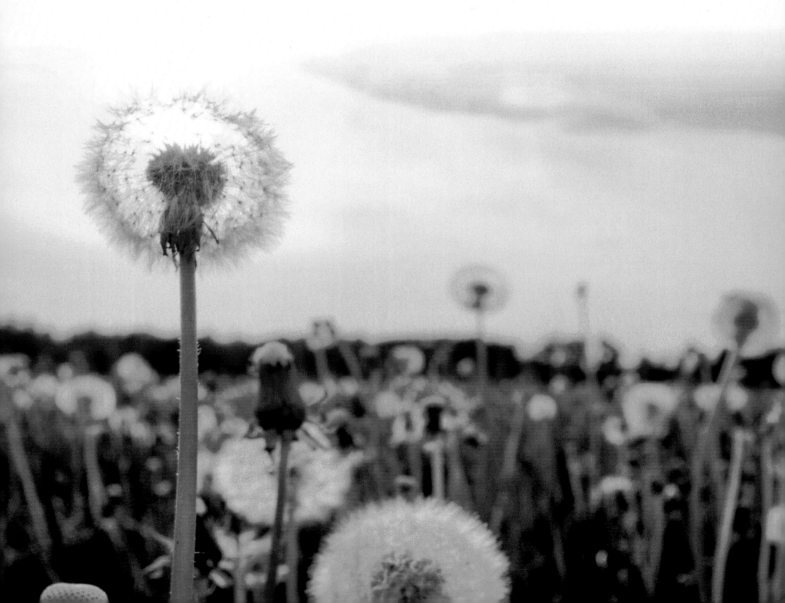

Your Heart's True Desires

Before you read any more of this book, I want to ask you a deep and profound question – a question so simple yet so potent that it has the power to totally transform your life.

Once you know the answer to this question, the deeper part of you will begin work all day and all night to provide you with answers and solutions to your challenges and get you on your way to the life you want.

The question is:

Are you willing to Explore YOUR HEART'S TRUE DESIRES?

Before you answer this question, I want you to know this is not just a book you have in your hands. This is an opportunity to completely transform your entire existence; and it all begins with you, right now, declaring what you truly desire. Just remember that you are what you spend your time and energy doing on a daily basis. You already have the deep, innate wisdom to know what is right for you.

You might want to do the following exercise at a park or in a café. You are going to visualize how you would choose to go forward in your life.

So what ARE your heart's true desires? You can find out by asking the following questions and tuning in to how your heart FEELS:

Imagine you had all the time and money you could ever need AND you had no fear.

- How would you experience the world around you?
- What would you LOVE to do that would make a difference in your life?
- Who would you be?
- Imagine someone describing your life or paying you a tribute as you transition into the nonphysical world.
- What is the person saying about you?
- How do you want to be remembered?
- What would you like to be remembered for?
- If you could only achieve ONE thing in your life, what would it be?
- What do you want others to say about you?
- What do you want them to say with respect to what you stood for?
- What did you accomplish?

What choices will you make about your life so that you will never have any regrets?

Yes, these are deep and profound questions, and they can be a little intimidating at first; but as you allow yourself to go deep and answer with your heart, you tap into the eternal magic of the universe that is hidden away in your heart.

Once your heart is set on something – a goal, a dream worth living and dying for – nothing can stop you. The world becomes your playground, and all things come together.

Let us remember that this is YOUR journey. This is YOUR book, and I am simply here to help you discover your own path to health, newness, and healing.

Take the time to ask these questions and let them activate your hidden powers. You may have already received answers just by asking once. If so, write the answers down and put them where you will see them often to remind you of and connect you with what you truly desire.

Many people will be unable to answer these questions quickly due to decades of being told what to do or living other people's desires. This is fine. Simply keep asking the question, for in the question lies the answer. It may come when you are nice and relaxed in the shower, when you are half asleep, or at a moment when you are singing your favorite song or watching a film that touches your heart. Be open to newness. Be open to listen and receive. As you become open, magic will happen!

There is no rush. There is no one right answer. All you need to do is ask the question and listen to your heart. You can trust your heart, your inner knowing. It will help you elevate your consciousness and enable you to change your concept of yourself. You may have been raised to be ordinary, but you can choose to change this self-concept by unlearning the ways in which you were taught to be ordinary. You can choose to do what you have always wanted to do.

As you follow through on the changes you want to make in your life, you will accelerate your healing process and live the best life ever.

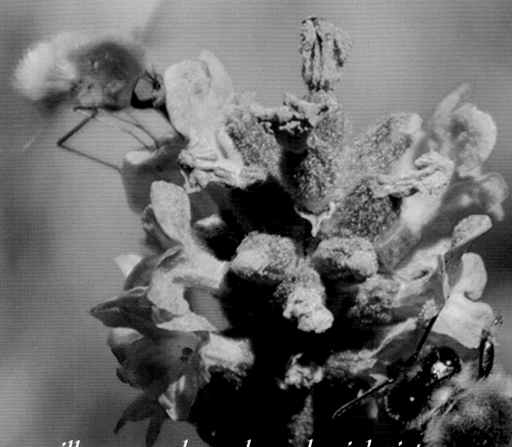

I feel certain there will come a day when physiologists, poets and philosophers will all speak the same language.

(Claude Bernard – physiologist – 1813-1878)

23

Models of Healing

Claude Bernard's quote very succinctly attests to the fact that health is not necessarily a domain in which only medical doctors can claim to have expertise. There are many models of healing apart from the medical model explained below. The discourse on the cause of dis-ease, in light of the complexities of the human body, points to the fact that dis-ease can spring from a multitude of roots: physical, emotional/psychological, spiritual, cultural, and environmental (Poole 1993). However, mainstream medicine, tends to address only the physical component. As Dr Deepak Chopra points out, all of western medical doctors' training is based on this mistake of the intellect.

Western Medicine

There is a general misconception that there is one type of medicine that is practised in Western medicine. In reality, each country treats illness differently based on their different cultural traditions. For example, if you were examined by a German doctor, the treatment protocol would most often be to strengthen the whole body, with a focus on the heart, as it is seen not only as a circulatory organ but as the seat of emotion.

The French too believe that all ailments are caused by internal weakness, but unlike the Germans, they are preoccupied with 'liver crisis' (*crise de foie*), and prescriptions often include tonics, vitamins, and spas to shore up the body's terrain (*le terrain*) that is in disequilibrium.

English medicine, like American medicine, has traditionally focused on external causes of disease and offers more antibiotics and other aggressive forms of pharmaceutical therapies to fight bacteria.

The doctor of the future will give no medicine but will interest his patients in the care of the human frame, in diet and in the cause and prevention of disease.

(Thomas A. Edison)

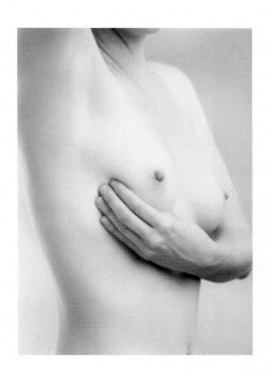

In some way which you know not of, through some process which never reveals its face,
Life has entered you and with it, the irresistible impulse to create:
Divine intelligence has willed it so…create or perish is the eternal mandate of
nature….
This thing seeks expression through everything – you may call it good or bad, right
or wrong, God or the devil, heaven or hell…Would it not be more simple to say that
finally things work out for the best only when they are life-giving.
You already are a spiritual being.
When the mind understands this and embodies its existence,
that which you are in the invisible will become more apparent in the visible.
Because you are created in the image of the one infinite creator, your desires…are
already here within you. The only things which stand between you and and it are
the conditioning/virtual reality of accumulated thoughts, beliefs and emotions of the
ages, your inherited tendencies and environment …These can be removed…..It is
futile to blame anything or anyone. Identify yourself with goodness, joy and straight
thinking…with faith. No one can give these to you but yourself and if you have them
no one can take them away from you.

(Ernest Holmes)

Eastern Medicine

As in Western medicine, there are many Eastern medical traditions, all of which are culture-specific. In the Indian medical philosophy, the root of all dis-ease is seen to lie in the concept of energy called *prana*. As the quotation on page 26 points out so eloquently, when the body's energy system is balanced, dis-ease is eliminated at its root. This is done through a holistic approach that aligns mind, body, and soul using meditation, diet protocols, and exercise movements such as yoga.

Like Indian medicine, Chinese medicine perceives that the cause of all disease lies in stuck energy or *chi*. Chinese medicine includes herbal, acupuncture, and diet protocols. Breathing and exercises in movements such as t'ai chi and Chi Gong are an integral part of this holistic medical philosophy.

I have written this book after ten years' of research in both Eastern and Western traditions, and what I have applied to myself through personal experimentation, and what I teach in my courses. It is a results-based approach. It has been proven beyond doubt that the human body is a self-healing mechanism. As Dr Ellie Drake points out in the quote (page 28), it is not a matter of fixing and curing with drugs. It is a process of recognising the root cause of the ailment and reintegrating this knowledge.

Healing is different from fixing and curing. It is a wholesome process of recognition and reintegration. Healing occurs when...

We release our negative dialogue and relationship to our body, mind and Spirit.

We release our negative relations to other people.

We realize that there really is no us and them, and that there is only us.

We realize the difference between self and Self, and

We bring back together any parts of us that have become separate from the whole.

(Dr. Ellie Drake – international spiritual and transformational speaker, entrepreneur)

This book gives you proven techniques, diet, and exercise protocols that activate our inherent biological processes so that the body can heal itself when it is properly taken care of at the level of mind, body, and spirit. It is my belief that I am obliged to share this information with you so that you can supercharge your health and live the best life ever.

I have deliberately chosen an eclectic approach to healing as I am interested in helping people rather than holding on to any rigid ideas and being "right." I am of the opinion that every individual is unique: what works for one person may not necessarily work for another.

Organisation of the book

This book consists of seven chapters.

In Chapter 1, I share my story with you.

In Chapter 2, I go into deeper reasons why you developed cancer and how to learn from them now to improve your life.

Chapter 3 focuses on your fears and frustrations about cancer and how you can overcome them.

Chapter 4 debunks myths around healing in mainstream medicine.

In Chapter 5, you are given the key to unlock the power of your mind.

Chapter 6 gives you several daily rituals from which you can choose those that resonate with you to create vibrant health and happiness.

In Chapter 7, I present cutting-edge nutrition that will enable you to enjoy optimal health by choice (and stay cancer-free).

Many other details are beyond the scope of this book, but I invite you to visit my website for more information:

newlifefterbreastcancer.com

I encourage you to share this information with your friends and family.

Thank You!

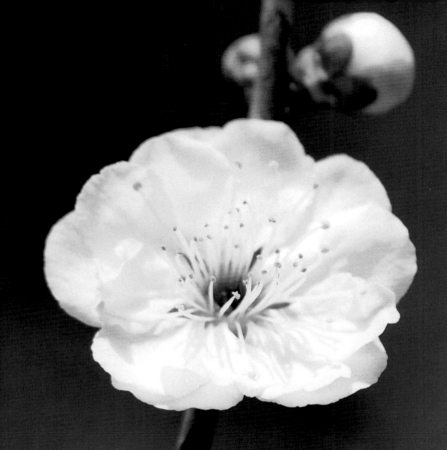

Everything is Energy. If you want to find the secrets of the universe, think in terms of energy, frequency and vibration.

(Nicola Tesla, inventor, engineer, futurist)

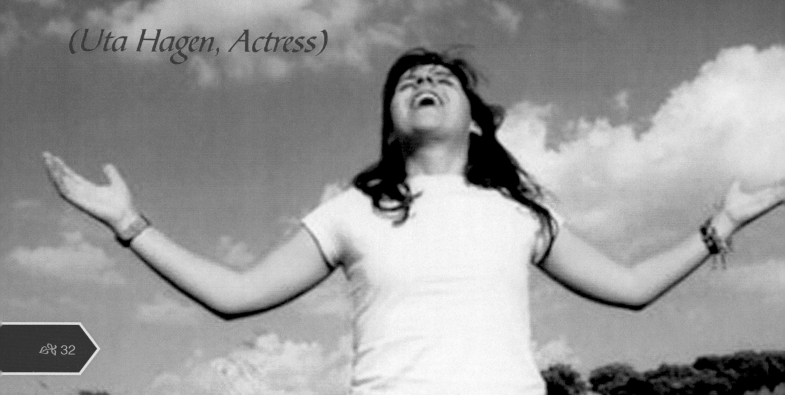

We must overcome the notion that we must be regular. It robs you of the chance to be extraordinary and leads you to the mediocre.

(Uta Hagen, Actress)

Chapter 1
My Story

The entire universe is a web of relationships that holds everything together. Entangled inside this web we create endless stories in our on-going movie (of life) and this movie is what we call the physical body and the physical world.

(Dr. Deepak Chopra)

We, humans, love a good story! We work and play with childlike imagination in this way – naturally. Our whole life is a series of short chapters. These real life movies depict many genres: Sci-Fi thrillers, romance, super boring soap operas (to say the least).

A part of my story includes my creation of a disease called cancer. Like any epic novel, there is an exciting prequel, a dark and challenging main series and a happy never-ending as life is eternal.

I now write this second edition of the Greatest Gift series as a deeper director-producer and protagonist to my challenging health story. Roles that emerged out of my transformation through self-realization. As Dr Michael Beckwith so wisely says, pain pushes us and our vision pulls us. For without a vision we perish, without a vision we founder, without a vision we fall. The Universe desires us to evolve and tap into our latent potential in the shortest possible "time" in the timeless Now.

My vision is to make an impact in the world through personal transformation. So in this book I will share some tools that I used to self-realize and empower myself to create a life worth living. A joyful, inspired life focussed on transcending the human condition and being one with my natural self/authentic self. Feeling grateful for every challenge that my natural self has sent me to fulfill this vision with a loving, compassionate heart.

This book is offered as a gift to my readers with the intention that humanity does not suffer needlessly in ignorance and fear of questioning decadent belief systems that keep us from unleashing our true potential. We live in a progressive universe that delights in replacing what no longer serves with newer creative insights. With hindsight, I know that cancer (amongst other challenges) has helped me create a life I now choose to live – new and fresh. Living moment by moment, following my highest excitement with childlike wonder.

It has been a unique journey, a unique life for we are all created uniquely. It is my desire that you too will embrace your uniqueness, and share your unique and wonderful gifts you have come to share with the rest of the universe. And simultaneously cease unnecessary suffering through traumas and dramas.

This book is my *gift* to you.

So, let's get started. As we dive deep into the theatre of life we may even re-write the script in light of new insights gleaned through meditation. Thank you for journeying as deeply as you are with the challenge. Every baby step benefits all of humanity in ways that defy both logic and imagination!

The scene is etched in my soul forever. I will never forget the day in 1997 about a week after I had triumphantly submitted my Ph.D. thesis. I had my flight booked to visit my mother and siblings in Kuala Lumpur, the city where I was born and raised – one of my favorite places.

However, I never boarded the plane. A few days before leaving I had felt a lump in one of my breasts and had to have a biopsy to check things out before I went on my holiday.

Little did I know when I walked into the clinically clean hospital that I would be confronted with the three most scary, devastating words I had ever heard: "You've got cancer." My heart stopped. My stomach rebelled. I have always considered myself physically fit and healthy (being the athletic sort). I felt that I was handling all life's difficulties well and everything seemed fine.

This was the most distressing and bewildering time of my life. As a new migrant, I had no family support in Australia and few friends. I had left my precious childhood friends behind when I chose to tread the path less trodden.

I felt vulnerable, so I handed over my life to the doctors as I had no thoughts of my own; I could not think straight. In fact, I had negative thoughts and feelings. I felt derailed. My mind was a fog of confused thoughts. I am sharing this so you will know that your body is going to store these feelings and trauma in every one of its cells until you do something post-surgery to remove them.

I was afraid I would lose my breast, and thoughts of how that would affect my future raced through my mind uncontrollably. When I asked the surgeon what the chances were, he replied, "I don't know." That made me even more scared.

As it turned out, I was lucky that it was a grade two tumor that did not require a mastectomy. However, my trauma was not over yet. The next thing I heard was that pathology indicated that the surgeon had made an error: he didn't quite excise the margins of the tumor and therefore he needed to cut out a little more tissue a week later. Needing more surgery was a double blow. This made me even more frustrated and fearful. I was back to square one, worrying about losing my breast; but this time I was assured that would not happen.

In those days, there was no way to test whether the cancer had spread to the lymph nodes, so I had a third round of surgery to remove some lymph nodes from my armpit as well. Luckily, they were all clear.

For a couple of days after these three operations I felt terribly depressed, as this scene of hospitals and physical pain was so foreign to me. When the surgeon came round the following morning, I asked if I could be discharged, and he allowed me to go home with a drain. When I came out of the hospital, I felt very weak. Although I had not died, I was not fully alive. These were horrible days. Despite taking six aspirin daily, the pain was unbearable. I was crying constantly as the aspirin became less and less effective. I felt powerless. Life didn't seem worth living.

The operations were followed by six weeks of toxic radiotherapy to ensure that any remaining "renegade" cancer cells would not multiply. Unfortunately, some of the surrounding healthy tissue too was also radiated.

The radiotherapy was not too bad, but it was an experience I would rather not have had as it led to other digestive challenges later on. Though I appreciated the visits from my colleagues and friends, I wanted the six weeks to pass swiftly. I was looking forward to going home and could not wait for a change of scenery. At times I felt as though my life was over. I didn't like the idea of having to be on guard for ten years and enduring painful mammograms yearly. The very thought of them made me feel "less than," incomplete. The numbness in my armpit was a constant reminder.

My breast was tender and inflamed. I had to buy new cotton brassieres without underwire that were not easy to find. I was wondering if I had to throw away my pretty, lacy Elle McPherson bras that were such a good fit for me! It is strange how such things affect you.

At the same time, I felt most appreciative of the medical profession for helping me through this crisis, especially to my world-renowned breast surgeon, despite his error. It is human to err. He was most loving and caring and was available 24/7 post-surgery.

What does this mean for you? If surgery is the only option, you need to seek the best possible medical experts in the world, as your health is your wealth.

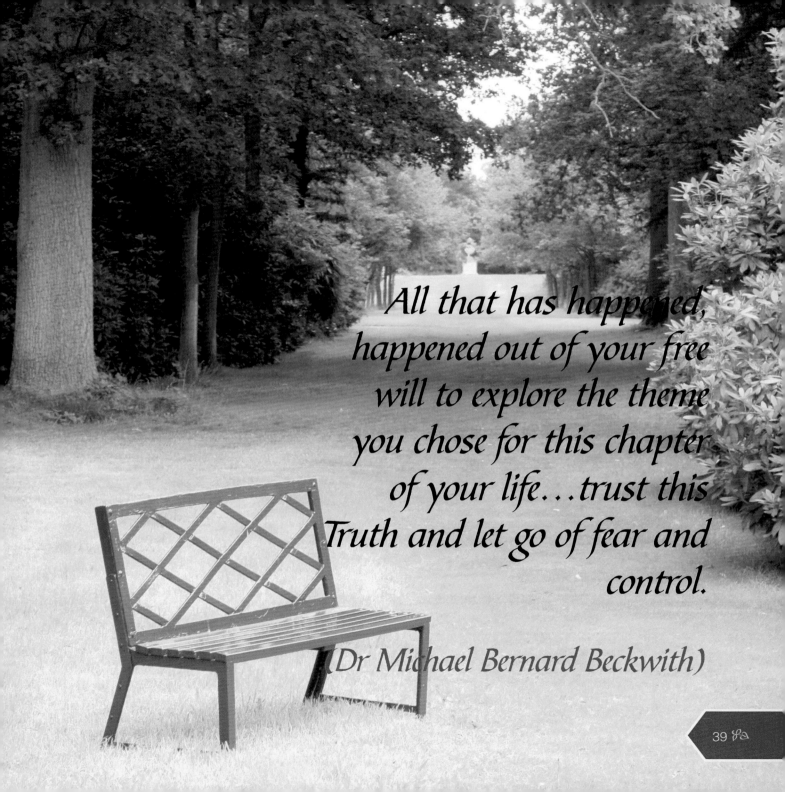

All that has happened, happened out of your free will to explore the theme you chose for this chapter of your life...trust this Truth and let go of fear and control.

(Dr Michael Bernard Beckwith)

My story after cancer and what I hope you will achieve too.

Once I got over the shock and depression, I began to ponder the cause of this traumatic, life-shattering experience; and it didn't take me too long to shed light on it. I had to turn the clock back 17 years to find the answer to this question. In subsequent years, I had to delve even more deeply beyond space and time. But more on this later.

Cancer is a disease that takes 15 to 20 years to manifest (Dr. Sangeeta Pati, Integrative Medicine Physician – interview with David Wolfe on BestDayEver.com, February 2012).

My first realization was that I had brought this disease upon myself through childhood patterns I had acquired. I traced the root cause to 1980 when I was living in Malaysia and chose to live my true nature by going against sociocultural

Don't be too quick to interpret the moment. Just keep quiet.

My encouragement would always be: never think anything is against you; everything is a blessing. Why should it be different?

Just be quiet. Let it all work itself out.

Mooji (Spiritual teacher, author, artist, visionary, public speaker)

To most people reading this book, this may seem both impossible and even unnecessary. Our education (especially western education and philosophy) compels us to rationalize and act Now! The advice of much psychology and mainstream medical profession would lean in this direction.

My "Greater Gifts" through faith healing and deeper energy work taught me the effects of negativity, playing the blame game, overthinking; figuring things out with the surface cognitive mind. The depth of my suffering taught me the more subtle effects in the momentum of the mind and the energetic relationship to the body. In addition, we are influenced by the energy of others in much the same way that the older crystal radio sets used to pick up the frequency of a radio station. This may seem radical to many people reading this, but in truth, both modern science and natural human observation shows us that there are energies of people (and other dark energies) constantly entangled in co-relation.

These unhealthy energies would be my greater gift in a deeper relationship with positive energies of the heart. The deeper bioelectric field described in recent science is delving into the spiritual practices of higher light or "star" frequency of pure consciousness. Many faiths describe this in different words: zen self, spirit, soul, source energy, Buddha self, Christ Consciousness or core existence. This is our real self that is pure love. As Dr Deepak Chopra and other visionaries have pointed out, healing is a return to this memory....You are not your body. You have the experience of a body. It is an activity of the Universe. And that activity is happening in you. In the deeper domain of existence there is only the real (unconditioned) you.

The 1980s were a time of career and relationships. It was also a time of being publicly exposed in the most private of things. It seems there was no sacred space for me in the bedroom or outside – this was the psychological terrorism of my private world. With hindsight, I have learned to be grateful for these betrayals – to allow them to come and to allow them to leave.

The backdrop of this story also unravels within a very conservative culture. It was not easy being a nonconformist in a culture that frowns upon sleeping with a man prior to marriage.

The first year was the hardest year to cope with. I had gained notoriety by choosing to be myself. Being under constant surveillance did not help my self-esteem. I began to develop a poor self-image, worrying that people would not like me for who I was.

Through the law of attraction (i.e., what we focus on we attract) I was unconsciously attracting the wrong partners into my life and co-creating negative experiences for myself. This is what happens if you are unhappy in your own skin, as I was unhappy because of the storms of persecution that I was going through. I began to feel unworthy while still determined to be who I was.

Many decades later, my gift is a deep surrender. A sweet surrender to my real self which is beyond the human fabrication of name, conditioning and personhood. When we no longer desire the outside circumstances to change, paradoxically, the outside will change too. The deeper healing comes from listening to the still small voice through spiritual practices. We learn that we are vibrational beings living in a vibrational universe. Becoming rooted in this Truth, knowing that only our state of being matters, we no longer take cues from external circumstances.

For many, reading this book, such a concept goes against every mental instinct instilled in us. However, the voice of experience now is in alignment with many people who have faith in the Truth that we create our reality.

I can't stress enough how important it is to create your own happiness (from within yourself). Be content with your internal approval and avoid looking for external validation. When you go against societal rules, you can expect resistance. Even though it is painful, irritating, and annoying, it is not fatal. On the contrary, it will only make you stronger, more emotionally resilient. With time, you will cease to look for outside validation and external approval. You will grow and evolve.

With this colorful experience behind me, I decided to make a fresh start by migrating to Australia in 1992 to complete my Ph.D. in Conversation Analysis. Though I had been warned that this "shadow" of persecution might follow me to my new home, I decided to migrate anyway, for I believed I would have a new beginning. I have a bright faith in human nature even during times of adversity.

Imagine my shock when a friend in Australia received a voice message suggesting I was an "imposter." My friend was puzzled why I was treated like a "terrorist." Another friend wanted to know how I was a threat to national security! Needless to say, these incidents brought on a new wave of paranoia, and I started to lose the ability to cope with my daily life.

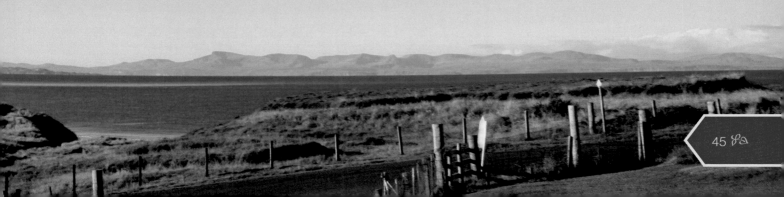

Dropping your fear of humiliation will strengthen your self-esteem. Humiliation is a choice, after all. When you stop the habit of looking for situations to be offended by, then you stop choosing to be humiliated. In addition, when you know and trust that everything that happens is constantly strengthening you, it follows naturally that you can be humble on the inside and bold on the outside, and grow through every step of the journey.

(Dr. Ellie Drake)

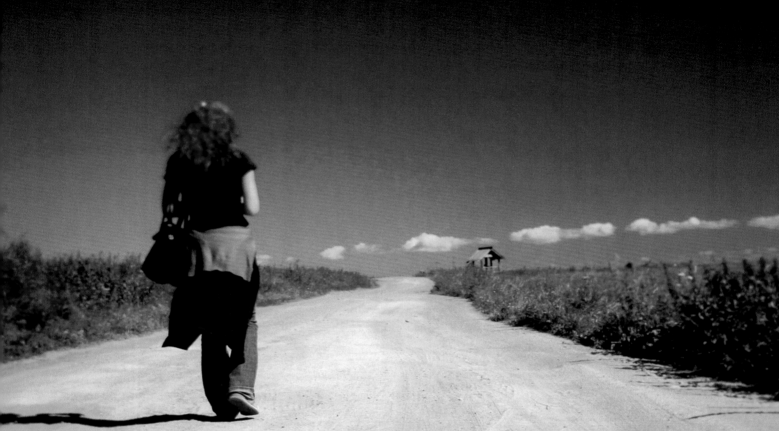

No one can hurt you today without triggering
a hurt from your past. You have to see that
in order to find yourself.

(Dr Deepak Chopra)

The Panic Attacks Started

And the story continues!

I began to have anxiety attacks. I was encouraged to take medication, but I soon realized that it was ruining my immune system and therefore ruining my life even more.

What does this mean for you? Medications do not help; they are just a band-aid solution. In fact, pharmaceutical drugs can do more harm than good to your brain chemistry. They treat your symptoms momentarily but not the root cause, which is your energetic patterns.

Talk therapy did not help either because the problem I was having was about my patterns – my energetic patterns – which is all about the right brain, my feelings.

It was around this time that I was diagnosed with breast cancer, which made things even worse. However, soon after my surgery I met my future husband, a lovely Italian academic who gave me much empathy and support. He helped me wash away some of my shame and helped me blossom again. I began to live in joy. Against doctors' orders, I weaned myself off the medications I was on. I learned not to react, to accept the "ugly things" that were going on, to learn to live without privacy, and to ignore the harassments.

How can you avoid going through such drama? Know that even though you may be in the eye of a storm, you can make a cognitive shift into joyful memories to ride the storm. Your freedom lies within you, but it takes courage to become self-aware. Awareness precedes action.

I lost some friends because of the harassment I was receiving, but I discovered that those who are your true friends will always stand by you through thick and thin. I wanted to live my truth and live a life that matters, no matter what. I wanted to make a difference in the world. I soon learned to embrace my challenges, for they made me stronger. And you can do the same. Challenges are actually gifts wrapped in sandpaper. They help us grow and experience evolution. I can't stress enough how important it is to honor your authentic self.

During this time I realized that I had developed unconscious patterns of feeling unloved, of feeling repressed and oppressed, of being persecuted, of being rejected. I began to feel insecure from time to time.

Unbelievably, just as I was grappling with these issues of self-confidence, I received yet another blow. I was diagnosed with early signs of cervical cancer. I was faced with two choices: to go back to conventional treatments or embrace an alternative medical solution. I chose the latter.

My physician, who practiced integrative medicine, put me on some supplements to deal with the condition nutritionally. It worked. I was living in London then and was on holiday for eight months. I believe the absence of the work pressures and daily stressors that I had been living with helped expedite my recovery too. I was out of the intensely crazy "war zone."

What does this mean for you? It means that you do not need to begin cutting yourself up at the first sign of danger; there are other therapies available to you. It also means that these symptoms are your body's way of talking to you, asking you to nurture yourself, love yourself, accept yourself, and value yourself – to wake up, re-examine your life, and become more of who you really are. This means that you have to embody self-love and self-appreciation.

An unexamined life is not worth living.

(Socrates)

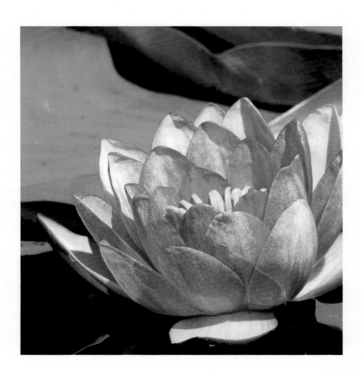

You are responsible for your life. You can't keep blaming somebody else for your dysfunction. Life is really about moving on.

(Oprah Winfrey – talk show host, actress, producer, philanthropist)

You can wake up from this (old) story. With fresh insights you can de-construct and re-create a new story. The range of human perception is infinite. because consciousness is infinite.

(Dr Michael Bernard Beckwith)

It wasn't until one morning in London in 2008, as I was taking a journey inward, that I had the realization that the real cure to cancer lay inside me. Dealing with what was inside of me was the only way I could get my life back. It dawned on me that I was living quite a powerless, limiting life; so I just woke up, metaphorically speaking.

This awakening was about consciousness bringing me back to the truth of who we truly are, our natural childlike state. The intensity of emotions was the guidance trigger to steer me back to the lighter vibrations when we are aligned to our true nature. Following our joy and passion helps us remove the mask of human identity, the conditioned self.

It is an extraordinary journey to overcome cancer both physically and emotionally. However, the Greater Gift would be delivered by a deeper challenge, both inwardly and outwardly around the world and within my being. I am so grateful for the many people and amazing locations that crossed my path. I was gathering more and more practical life tools for the further deeper challenges to come. My travels took me to the most well known people in natural health on almost every continent.

It was upon my return to Australia that this depth of psychological and energetic terror met me in full force. It was the Christmas and New Year period of 2016 to 2017 when I was 'admitted'. It is somewhat ironic that people forming my close relationships who are also technically colleagues with their own doctorates and PhDs in the field of medicine or psychology should wish to have me 'admitted' in a psychiatric ward and inject me with drugs against my free will. From those that know me, or read my work outside this field of work would naturally be most surprised . Nevertheless, when working deeply in the field of complementary medicine or natural medicine, the depth of the challenge is met with the most extreme protagonist in the 'real life' movie.

And so from the inside of the 'ward' I can share deeper and more profound realizations. I share this with you so that you can use the tools and insights I have to offer without having to go through such an extreme terror of a movie. The scope of this book is too deep and profound for just one book and so I will shortly leave this particular 'scene' of the story so that I can share more of the real life application of Cancer's Greatest Gift.

What I would like to share at this stage of the series is that being on the 'inside' of a psychiatric ward, and then doing this depth of healing to share in joy and happiness on the outside is that you can easily apply the principles I am about to share without such an extreme movie plot! In future books in the series, there will be more terror scenes and even more happy never endings! Terror movies can be very stimulating but are best avoided if you can!

As there is much to say in the lead up to the following chapters of helpful health and wellbeing tips, I would like to say that these 'so called' energies I spoke of earlier are quite unhealthy in their nature due to our conditioning to block our sensitivity of them. It is well known of the unhealthy energies emitted by mobile phones and their towers. However, there more subtle energies that can hijack our minds. These are interesting times for awakening and taking our minds back!

And so, enough of the terror scenes in my life story, let's move on to thinner joy, love and radiant health to which we all aspire! Thank you for being radiant, loving and enjoying real aliveness with m through our challenges. Let's re-write our script together in these coming chapters!

The Big Change: How My Life Started to Turn Around for the Better

I soon recognized that I required change, an inner change. I learned and practiced Tapping and Quantum Energy Transformation (I explain these in Chapter 5) – two extremely powerful alternative healing modalities that have helped me remove all the traumas that had been frozen in the cellular memories of my body. I consider them far superior to talk therapy as they are body-based, right-brain healing modalities that helped release my essence as I began clearing my emotional and psychological clutter.

I also engaged some of the best therapists in the world. They were highly intuitive, for they had done their own inner work. This is the beauty of alternative therapies – these therapists can tap into their intuitive powers rather than just follow some theoretical flow chart/framework, which often leads to a wrong diagnosis.

What does this mean for you? You must give yourself the opportunity to seek alternative therapies that help you discover the CAUSE of your ailment rather than just rely on mainstream medicine because not many doctors go beyond the symptom to discover the cause. You do have a choice about treatment options.

I soon began to feel a sense of renewal and empowerment. I felt good experiencing this change; everything was coming together. I began to feel that everything happened for some celestial reason that was directed toward my enlightenment. I began to like who I was and who I was becoming. My energy levels doubled. I began to blossom personally, little by little. Now I feel grounded most of the time, and I am becoming an embodiment of love, light, and laughter as a result of it.

I hope you can benefit from these things I have learned on my healing journey thus far:

- I avoided playing the blame game and took 100 per cent responsibility for all that happened to me.

- I learned the importance of forgiveness and *letting go* of resentments. I learned that forgiveness is a visceral experience, not a mental one – that when you forgive, you forgive yourself first for living a less-than-optimal life, for not taking 100 per cent responsibility for all your actions and reactions. In this space you do not need to beat yourself up for being "less than." Instead, you embrace all your feelings and in so doing you release them and move forward.

- I changed my story and gradually created a new template for my evolution. I became emotionally resilient. I decided that I am not my reputation. It's my spiritual dignity that matters to me, and what others think of me is none of my business. Happy people have no time to judge others, so why should you be seeking the validation of someone who does not know the art of happiness in the first place?

- By seeing a doctor who practiced nutrition medicine, I learned the art of nutrition and how important nutrition is to one's health and well-being.

Our stories are a product of the human condition that causes so much suffering. The 5 main causes of suffering, as eloquently summarized by Dr Deepak Chopra are:

1. Not knowing the true nature of reality: Who Am I? You cannot be your body as it keeps changing. Nor your mind as your thoughts keep flickering to where you put your attention on. So Who Am I is the perennial question. Not knowing the answer creates a lot of suffering.

2. Clinging and holding onto that which is not real. If everything is a process (i.e., continually moving, shifting, transforming, flickering …) what is there to hold onto? Yet we are grasping: not letting go of what is keeping us stuck and embracing the evolutionary impulses that make us feel good.

3. Egoic structures rooted in fear of constant change and transformation.

4. The constricted/limiting identity we call our name and the meanings we associate with it.

5. Fear of death as we get attached to our physical life. But who dies? It's interesting that ancient wisdom traditions had a clue: that who you really are is nothing conceivable, imaginable or graspable. It's formless, changeless and has no height or width, no depth, no location, has no space, is timeless. Yet consciousness (our real self) remains unseen but without it there's no seeing. It remains unheard but without it there's no hearing. It remains untouched, untasted and can't be smelled, but without it there's no perceptual experience. What dies is what never was. Because there is no such thing as a thing: there's only a process in the unimaginable, inconceivable, formless ground of Being. And we are That. This is your true Self in the field of infinite possibilities in the Universe.

- I learned how to create self-love rather than looking for love outside of myself. I learned to grow and become more. I made my life juicy!

- I took up yoga and learned the importance of mind–body–spirit connection.

- I began rebounding and dubbed it the best exercise in the world!

- I gave up my academic career. (I had climbed the wrong mountain!)

- I began to see the significance of new experiences on my travels and broadened my horizons.

- I realized the importance of doing things that brought me joy, such as gardening and nature walks, as nature reflects our inner nature.

- I became aware that it is wise to invest in yourself, to engage the services of some of the best life coaches in the world for help and guidance in transforming your life.

- I learned to love my own company and to appreciate myself and others unconditionally. Through this trial-and-success method, I have created a new inner self-image.

Over the last 2 years I have been living a Breatharian lifestyle after dry fasting for up to 3 days at a time. I have re-set my body to a point where I now eat for the pleasure of eating. Anything is possible once we uncondition our conditioned minds.

What is new and different about me now?

- I put myself first; I fill my cup and others get to enjoy the overflow.
- I have changed my perception of who I am, making a life-changing paradigm shift.
- I know that I am a spiritual being having a temporary human experience.
- I have a nice relationship with myself (the most important relationship in my life) and others.
- I have expanded my perspectives on life and have become more open-minded and flexible, ever so open to trying new approaches to things in my life.
- Since I love myself, I live a fear-free life that is full of peace and joy most of the time.
- I have never felt healthier or more beautiful than I do now because I love my life and I love myself.
- I have a healthy sense of self-worth, self-respect, and self-love/acceptance.

- I am doing what I love and I love what I do – empowering women like you who have been through breast cancer so that you too can go on and live the best life ever.
- I am doing my bit in helping correct what has gone wrong with the world that is leaving people disempowered and lacking in self-love.

It is my desire that this book will help you live a life that is:

- happier and free of fear;
- healthier and free of pain;
- worth living and blessed with longevity;
- one in which you will feel good and look great;
- one in which you will easily keep your brain young and sharp;
- one in which you will maintain your perfect weight;
- one in which you foster the attitude that breast cancer has helped you solve a problem that your psyche could not figure out how to resolve, as this attitude will help you heal much faster.

To learn more about how I overcame my challenges, please visit my website:

newlifeafterbreastcancer.com

and feel free to pass this information to your friends and family.

Thank You!

He who lives in harmony with himself lives in harmony with the Universe.

(Marcus Aurelius, Roman Emperor)

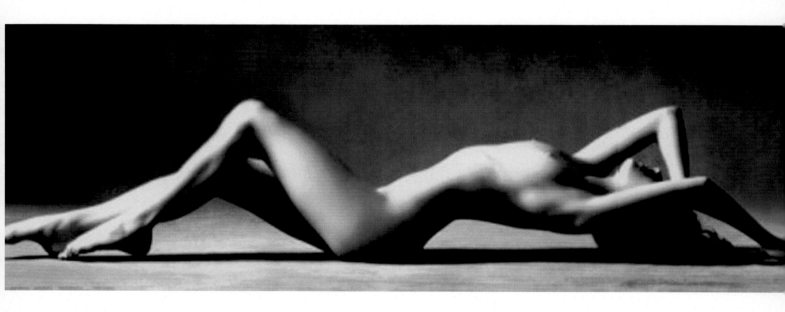

The body is the servant of the mind . . . .
At the bidding of unlawful thoughts,
the body sinks rapidly into disease and decay;
at the command of glad and beautiful thoughts it
becomes clothed with youthfulness and beauty . . . .
ease and health, like circumstances,
are rooted in thought. Sickly thoughts will express
themselves through a sickly body . . . .
Anxiety quickly demoralizes the whole body,
and lays it open to the entrance of disease;
while impure thoughts, even if not physically
indulged, will soon shatter the nervous system.

(James Allen, Author)

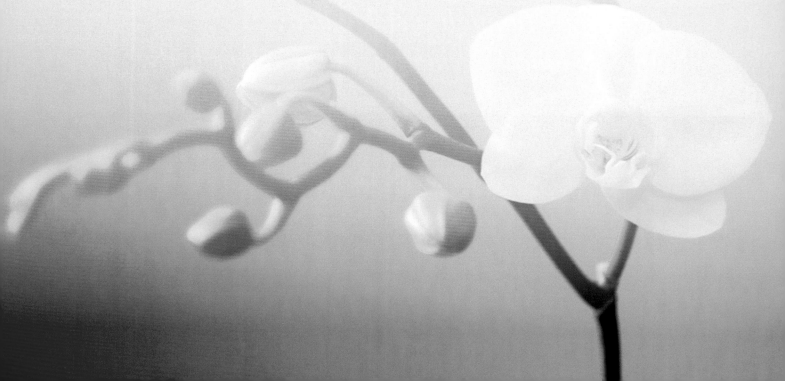

Chapter 2

Deeper Reasons on Why You Developed Breast Cancer and How to Learn from them Now to Improve Your Life

Why do some women develop breast cancer while others do not? It is a well-known phenomenon that people begin to enjoy life *more* after near-death experiences – they often turn their life around after such experiences.

Here is how you can turn your life around too. In this chapter, you will learn:

- what personality types are more prone to developing breast cancer;

- what psycho-emotional factors are common to most breast-cancer patients;

- how you can change your mindset and live a life free of fears of a relapse.

After seeing thousands of patients, cancer therapists have suggested many possible reasons for the development of cancer. For example, it is well documented that breast-cancer patients exhibit certain personality traits – your inner reality creates your outer circumstances.

Below are some positive characteristics you may be able to identify with:

- You are a nice person. You seldom complain, doing everything in your power to please everyone around you.

- You are extremely loving, caring, and giving.

- You are compassionate.

- You are generous and always strive to do the right thing by others.

- You tend to stay superficial in order to avoid arguments and conflict.

What You Can Do About It

Perfect health is your natural state. Disease / ailments are just symptoms your emotional guidance system is indicating that you are out of alignment with your natural state of being which is pure joy. When you feel vibrant and joyful, your emotional guidance system is telling you that you are in alignment with your authentic self. When you don't feel good, your emotional guidance system is telling you that you are out of alignment. Once you become aware of this Truth – that perfect health is your natural state – this awareness or consciousness will naturally begin to heal you. With this fresh insight, you will be inspired to transform your life by following some of the suggestions below that resonate with you.

1. Unlearn the automatic assumptions conditioned into you by your parents and society at large. The state of your body is intrinsically an indicator of your thought patterns indicating whether (a) you are living in alignment with who you really are and consequently, (b) living in alignment with who or what you really love being and/doing. As all ailments are a result of misaligned thought, you can transcend thoughts and be one with your true self that awakens your spirit of wonder. However, there are some rare exceptions. As Bentinho Massaro points out, we may choose certain disabilities at a soul level – either we are born with them physically or we develop them over time, because we know that they are going to facilitate particular lessons or otherwise we would not go in the direction of learning them, moving in certain directions of thought and exploring life if we did not include these seeming limitations.

2. Re-consider your lifestyle. Are you pursuing a career path that is your parents' fantasy or are you exploring your theme, what you are meant to do by your true nature. Are you enjoying your "work" most of the time?

3. Reflect on your relationships with the people in your life. As your awareness of your true nature expands, you will realize that all relationships are a man-made fabrication, a human construct. Therefore you might begin to perceive your relationships in a way that are in alignment with your true self. For example, you would choose to spend more time on perfecting your own relationship with yourself for that is the only real relationship: your conditioned physical self and your unconditioned nonphysical true Self or what some might call your inner being. How you see life needs to be in alignment with who you really are. If you are not in alignment with how life actually works based on who you really are, then you begin to feed this misalignment into your body. Frequent negative thoughts are the first indicators of misalignment.

Love is always bestowed as a gift – freely,
willingly, and without expectation.
We don't love to be loved;
we love to love.

(Leo Buscaglia, Spiritual Author)

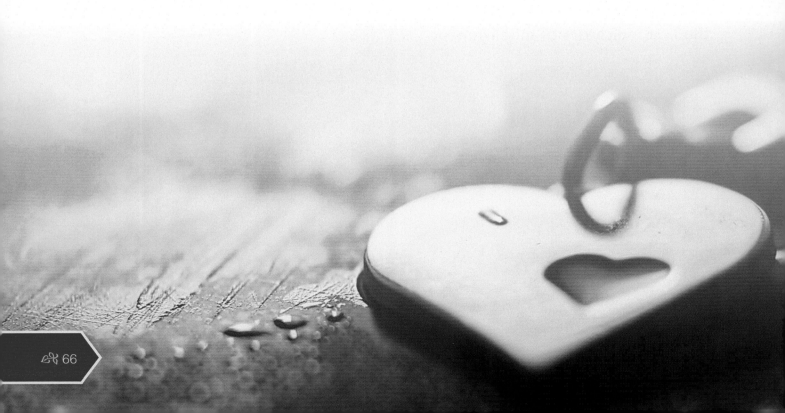

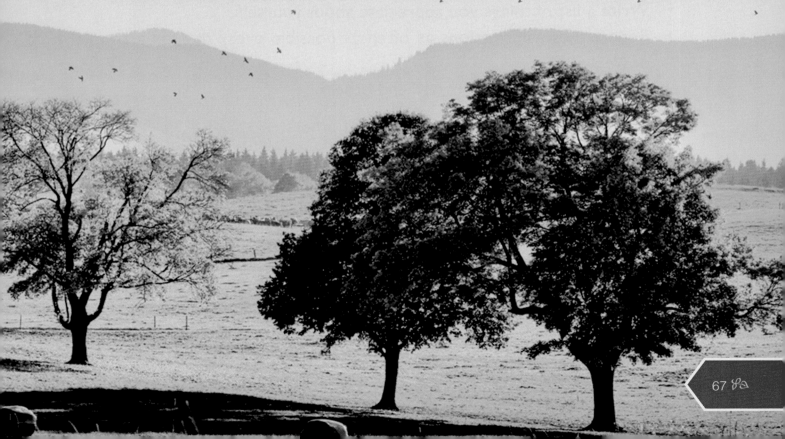

Joy is what happens when we allow ourselves to recognize how good things really are.

(Marianne Williamson – author, speaker, spiritual entrepreneur)

What You Can Do About It

You can restore the severed, sacred bond with yourself and raise your level of consciousness by doing the following:

- Release all negative self-talk about yourself (e.g., "I'm not good enough") and others by observing your thoughts. When we observe, we release the burden.
- Release the energy of low self-worth through oxy-breathing (see Chapter 5) and express your value through self-trust.
- Forgive yourself for being hard on yourself and for judging others.
- Write a list of things you appreciate about yourself.
- Repeat these affirmations as often as possible every day for a couple of weeks:

I release all judgments about myself and others.

I unconditionally love and accept myself and others.

Right now I am a whole, complete woman. (Luxuriate in this statement.)

Then consciously work on developing a new inner self-image. (See Chapter 5 for details on how to do this.) Be unafraid of pushing yourself beyond your comfort zone, creating a new comfort zone each time you make a subtle shift.

As you restore the bond between your body and your soul, you will begin your journey of true healing. You will become new and fresh.

To re-align yourself, ask yourself the following questions:

- How have I been bottling up my anger/aggression in order to be nice? (Being nice is a fantastic trait, but at what expense?)
- How have I cluttered my body with feelings of shame, fear, anxiety, and guilt? How is my relationship with my significant other/partner/husband going? Is there mutual trust?
- Where do I spend most of my energy – on things that make me more (e.g., self-nurturing) or on caring for others?
- Who are the six people I hang out with the most? Are they positive people? Do they uplift me? Do they inspire me to be who I really want to be, or are they controlling and manipulative?
- Am I controlling and manipulative? (If so, then my heart is closed and I am trying to protect myself.) Why can't I receive love/why don't I allow others to love me? What are my fears?

Perhaps it is time to go within and make a list of all the little events in your life that deeply hurt you. You will probably find that you can easily make a list of 100–150 events in your life that have been upsetting on the continuum of mildly depressing on one end of the scale to highly traumatic on the other end. Revisit those events one at a time, feel those feelings, and release them using the following breath technique:

Think of the hurtful event, feel the feeling, then take a deep breath. On the exhale, see yourself letting go of that event and the accompanying feeling. Then say "peace" within your heart.

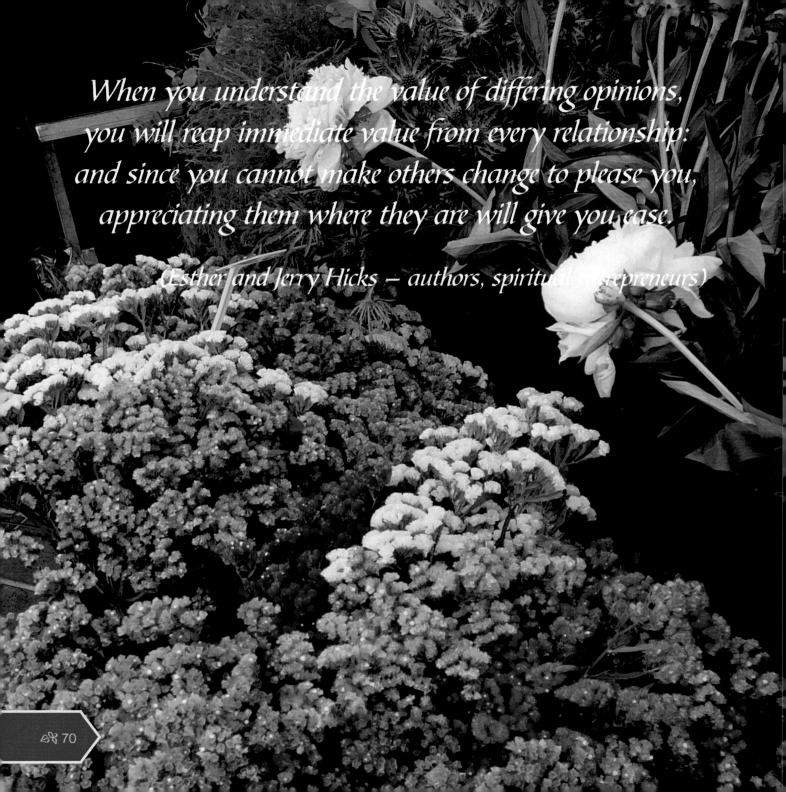

When you understand the value of differing opinions,
you will reap immediate value from every relationship:
and since you cannot make others change to please you,
appreciating them where they are will give you ease.

(Esther and Jerry Hicks — authors, spiritual entrepreneurs)

New Inner Self-Image Reminder

- Release all negative self-talk about yourself and others. (See Chapter 5.)

- Write a list of things you appreciate about yourself.

- Forgive yourself for feeling "less than" (e.g., "I'm not good enough, pretty enough," etc.).

- Forgive others who may have hurt you. Every person you forgive adds to your self-love. (See Appendix D.)

- Repeat the following affirmations as often as possible every day for a couple of weeks:

I release all judgments about myself and others.

I unconditionally love and accept myself and others.

Right now I am a whole, complete woman.

Pain pushes you - until your vision pulls you. You will be pushed by the universe to grow, often through painful measures, until you surrender to the higher vibration that is seeking to evolve through you.

(Dr Rev. Michael Beckworth, Founder of Agape International Spiritual Center, Los Angeles)

Work on creating a new inner self-image – What will you look like? How will you feel? What will you see? What will you be wearing? What will you be doing? What will you be touching? What will you be tasting? Emotionalize the new you into being.

For more information, please visit my website at

newlifeafterbreastcancer.com

to register for the weekly Live Events with Q & A, which will cover many more topics that could not be handled here due to space limitations.

I'd also appreciate it if you would share this vital information with your friends and family.

Thank You!

Fears are normal. It's the 'why' behind the fear that is a lie.

(Dr Guy Finley)

Neither a lofty degree of intelligence, nor imagination, nor both together go to the making of genius. Love, love, love: that is the soul of the genius.

(Wolfgang Armadeus Mozart)

Chapter 3

How to Overcome Your Fears and Frustrations About Cancer

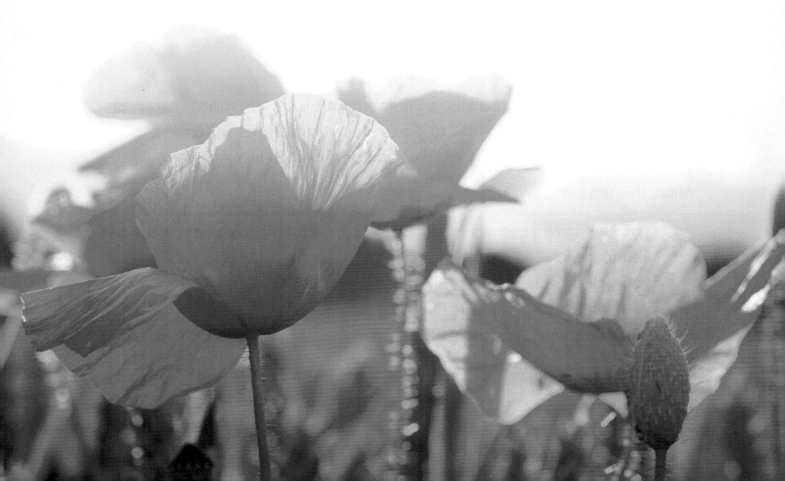

When you live from a place of fear, it is not possible for you to heal. On the contrary, you attract more and more health issues, for your body cannot thrive in this emotional state. In the long term, your immune system will be depressed, causing many other auto-immune problems.

Therefore, if you want to recover fully, avoid relapse, and have the best life ever, it is essential to overcome your fears. In fact, your fears may have been a major contribution to your having cancer in the first place because you had been suppressing your emotions for fear of rejection (or ridicule or disapproval). Perhaps you may not have been releasing your anger and resentments because you did not know how to do so. Living with fears (and thereby focusing on what you don't want) only makes matters worse.

In this chapter, you will learn:

- how to turn *fear* into *love of life* (and start living life more than ever);
- the main fears, and what to do to free yourself from them;
- how to rediscover the wonder and possibilities in your life

What this means for you is:

- you will love your way into optimal health and experience the joy of abundant, child-like energy;
- you will be able to enjoy life more;
- you will live an authentic life by being yourself;
- you will establish authentic boundaries for yourself.

How To Turn Fear Into Love of Life

Fear and love are mutually exclusive states of emotion. (Dr. Bruce Lipton, Dr. Wayne Dyer) It is impossible to love yourself, your life, or anyone if you are riddled with fears of this, that, and the other. Turning fear into love has to start with you. You need to get in touch with your essence and feel complete/whole in yourself so that you can then start living your life fully. When you know who you really are and that you are being your authentic self, you will then be able to live a life of your choosing. You will live a life that is fear-free and full of the love of life. Love heals.

Below are three steps you can take to be in your essence:

- Be true to yourself. Be authentic. Release all your emotional baggage: your fears and insecurities, your jealousies, your need to feel "less than," and your need for competitiveness. (See Chapter 5 for how to do this.)

- Live your life from a place of love and soul, not from your ego or lower self. (See Chapter 5 for details on how to do this.)

- Live in compassion, gratitude, and forgiveness of self and others. (See Appendix D on forgiveness.)

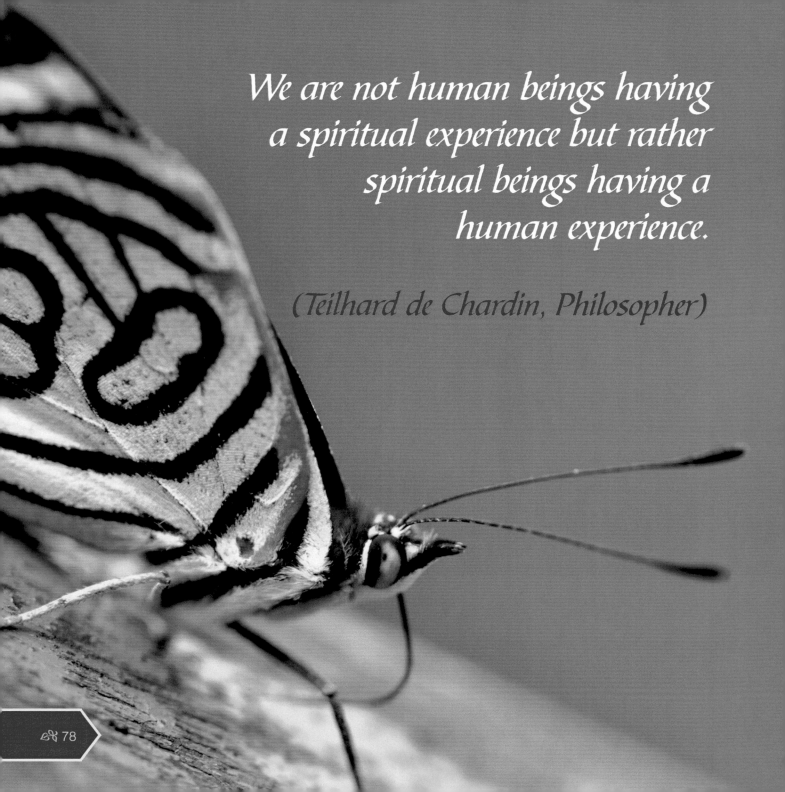

We are not human beings having a spiritual experience but rather spiritual beings having a human experience.

(Teilhard de Chardin, Philosopher)

Fear Number 1: The Fear of Death

The fear of death is a very normal, human fear to have in response to a cancer diagnosis because you have been programmed to believe there is no cure for it and thus cancer equals death. You may have heard of stories where women did die, perhaps due to metastasis, in which the cancer spread to the entire body in women who did not take action to deal with their health issues in time. Even in such advanced cases, alternative healing modalities have been proven to be effective if the patient is determined to heal and live.

To turn this fear around, follow these three steps:

- Tell yourself that you are birthless and deathless. As the quote on page 74 points out, you are an eternal/spiritual being having a human experience. When you "die," you will merely move out of this physical world into the non-physical, like moving from one room into another.

- Overcome this fear by shifting your energetic frequency; for example, when you feel this fear, observe it until you can release it and then change your thought pattern. Think of a time in your life when you felt most alive, when you felt you truly loved your life. Keep expanding on this feeling and anchor it in.

- Repeat this process each time you have fearful thoughts, and your fears should become weaker. Replace your fears with love, pure love. Love yourself – love your body exactly as it is, remembering that "when you change the way you look at things, the things you look at change." (Dr. Wayne Dyer) It's about aligning your conscious mind with your subconscious mind.

If these steps do not work for you, talk to an expert who can help you work through your fear.

There was a child went forth every day,
And the first object he looked upon and received with
Wonder or pity or dread, that object he became,
And that object became part of him for the
Day or a certain part of the day…
Or for many years or stretching cycles of years.

(Walt Whitman – American poet, essayist, journalist)

Fear Number 2: You Might Lose Your Breast

This fear too is natural, since your breasts may contribute significantly to your sense of femininity, your beauty-consciousness, and your self-image and may impact your sense of aesthetics. If you have had breast surgery and/or radiotherapy or chemotherapy, the chances of a relapse and hence the need to remove the whole breast are minimized, but you still need to take the necessary action steps to upgrade your life so that you do not live in constant fear.

If you have chosen not to have surgery and opt instead to heal yourself using alternative medicine with the supervision of an expert, you are usually healed (physically) when you can no longer feel the lump. However, you may still have fears of a relapse and of losing a breast.

To turn this around, here are three things you can do:

- Move out of your head and into your body by focusing your attention at the base of your spine. Breathe (healing energy) into the breast that is giving you some concerns. With practice, this should help you shift out of your fear-consciousness. If you are still afraid, you may want to have a scan or a mammogram yearly until you feel safe.
- When you have the "all clear" sign, take the necessary action steps to make radical, positive lifestyle changes. (See Chapter 6 on how to do this.)
- Supercharge your health by getting your nutrition in balance. (See the details on how to accomplish this in Chapter 7.)

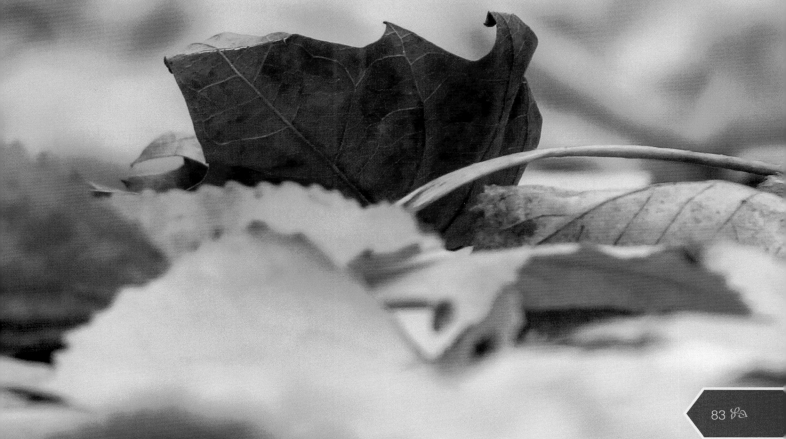

You can focus on what you see or you can focus on the Seer. You can focus on what you know or you can focus on the Knower.

(Bentinho Massaro)

Fear Number 3: I Don't Feel Attractive and/or My Partner or Husband Does Not Find Me Attractive Any More

After surgery, it is not uncommon to mentally and visually compare your breasts – the before picture being the more preferred one. You become self-critical, beating yourself up for all your health problems and feeling "less than" or "not enough" or perhaps feeling sorry for yourself.

Here are three steps to turn this around:

- Do the full-size mirror work where you appreciate yourself exactly as you are, releasing the negative feelings as they surface. (See Chapter 5 for details on how to do this.)

- When you have released the negative emotions, write a list of ten things you most appreciate about your body.

- Affirm: I love and accept my body exactly as it is. Repeat this affirmation until you begin to feel the truth of the statement and start to feel attractive again. Then you may add a more powerful affirmation such as I AM pure love. Repeat these affirmations just before you fall asleep so that the positive conscious thoughts will align with your subconscious mind.

When you change the way you look at things, the things you look at change.

(Dr. Wayne Dyer)

Fear Number 4: I Am Losing My Libido

Surgery can leave you feeling depressed, which in turn can lead to a loss of libido. As you may already know, your sexual desires always begin with thoughts in your mind. Your inner thought patterns of not being attractive, along with your fears, can lead to even more loss of libido with time. This can be a frustrating, vicious cycle, which can lead you to fall out of love with yourself and begin seeking love in the outer world of food or becoming too needy.

To turn this around, follow these three steps:

- See a qualified health professional practicing integrative medicine (which combines natural medicine with modern science), who will be able to advise you on your hormonal health and fire up your libido.

- Get your nutrition in balance. (See Chapter 7.)

- Exercise, as it restores your energy. (See Chapter 6.) It will give you muscle tone and help you like your body more.

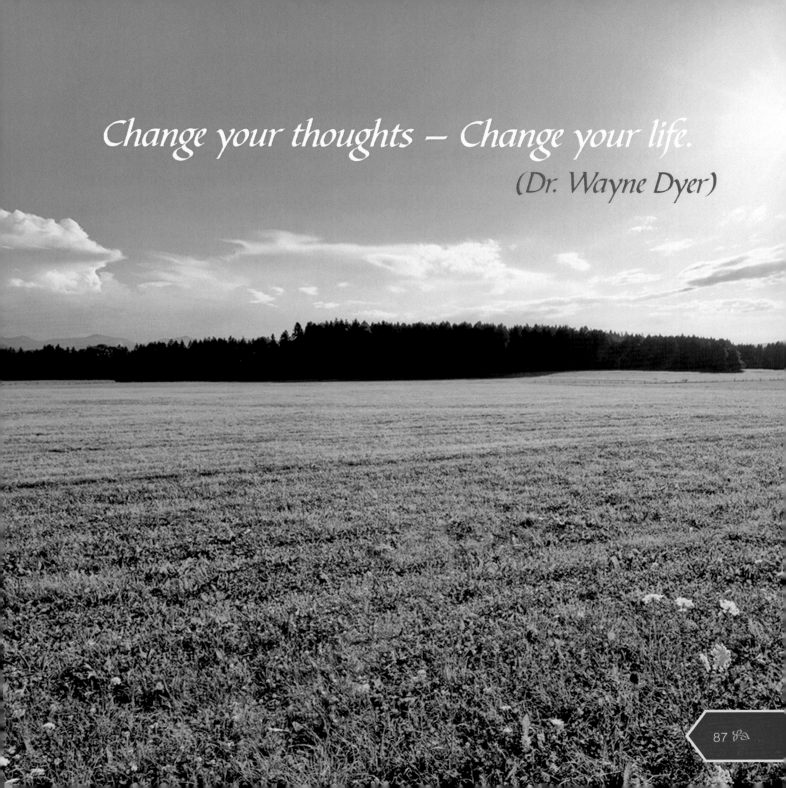

Change your thoughts – Change your life.

(Dr. Wayne Dyer)

Fear Number 5: I Am Not As Mentally Alert As I Used To Be (I Don't Know If I Can Handle All the Stress at Work)

It is not uncommon for you to feel that your brain is not working as well as it used to because of all the stress and shock you experienced when you discovered that you had breast cancer, coupled with your ongoing fears over a prolonged time. You will feel disempowered by the sheer weight of all that stress and trauma that may still be banging around in your system. However, this is also a common complaint among most women in today's fast-paced world. As mothers or even as single women, we do take on a lot of responsibilities.

To reclaim your brain and the power of your mind, take these three action steps:

- Get your lifestyle in balance. (See Chapter 6.)
- Get your nutrition in balance. (See Chapter 7.)
- Work on your psychological and emotional issues around stress, fears, and trauma (e.g., through healing modalities such as tapping, oxy-breathing, and quantum transformation). (See the details in Chapter 5.)

Now take a moment and ask yourself: *What are my biggest fears?* Each day of the week, work on embracing one fear and release it by doing this exercise:

Take a deep breath. On the exhale, visualize your fears leaving your mind and body, letting them go like clouds in the sky. As you release the fears, you will naturally allow love to flow into your life.

Love unlocks the heart, and gratitude bathes it in clarity. Together, Infinite Love and Gratitude are catalysts for extraordinary transformation, setting your spirit free.

(Dr. Darren Weissman – physician, author, lecturer)

If this does not work for you, refer to the tapping script in Appendix A and tap along to release your fears. Keep tapping as many times as possible for as long as it takes, until you are bored rigid! From my experience, shifts can happen in an instant or they may take up to a week.

As you go to bed, repeat these mantras:

I am perfect health.

I love and accept myself, no matter what.

As you flow through your day, keep saying these mantras as often as you can, preferably on the hour. Assume the feelings of these mantras from you heart. Always remember that as you change the way you look at things, the things you look at will change. So choose to focus on what you want. Choose to look for good-feeling thoughts.

For more information, please visit my website:

newlifeafterbreastcancer.com

and claim your *bonus: Secrets to Re-creating Life After Breast Cancer,* a three-part video series with downloadable materials.

"Fear-Free Life" Reminder To Rediscover the Wonder and Possibilities in Your Life

- See a nutrition expert you can trust to get your nutrition in balance.
- Get your lifestyle in balance – mix with people you resonate with, get enough exercise, get enough sleep, learn a little, laugh a little, and reflect a little each day.
- Work on your psychological issues – do breathing exercises and/or tapping to release your fears.
- Work on your spiritual issues – meditate; do yoga or a similar relaxing exercise.
- Discover your purpose in life – your service will bring joy to you and all around you.
- Live in your essence – be your authentic self. Do not pretend to be anything other.
- Repeat the mantras: I am perfect health.

    I love and accept myself, no matter what.

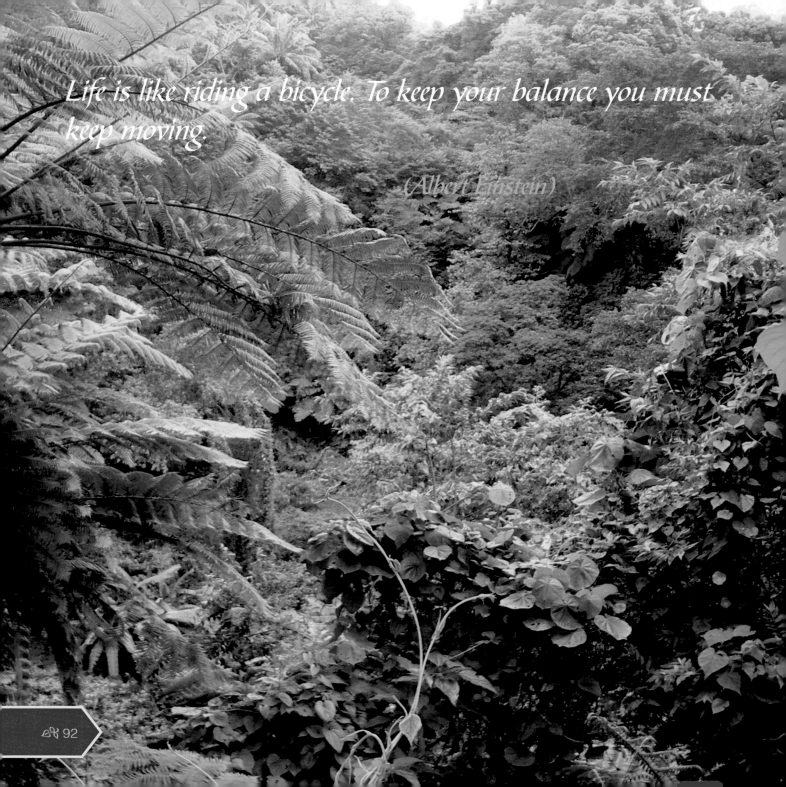

Life is like riding a bicycle. To keep your balance you must keep moving.

(Albert Einstein)

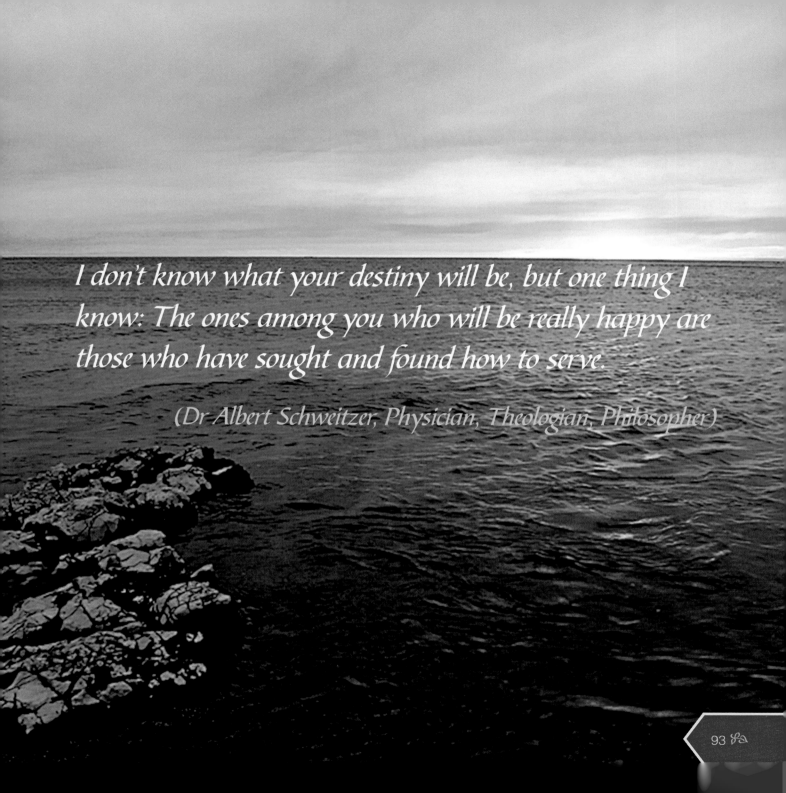

I don't know what your destiny will be, but one thing I know: The ones among you who will be really happy are those who have sought and found how to serve.

(Dr Albert Schweitzer, Physician, Theologian, Philosopher)

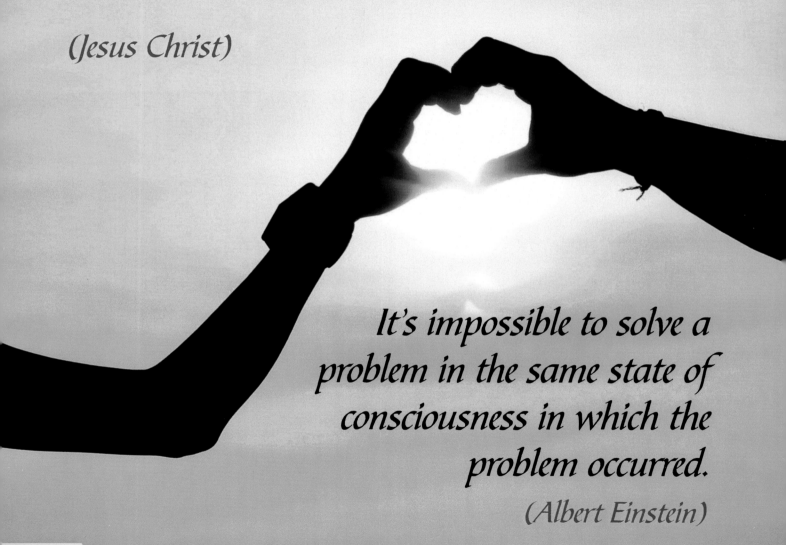

Perfect love casts out all fear.

(Jesus Christ)

It's impossible to solve a
problem in the same state of
consciousness in which the
problem occurred.

(Albert Einstein)

Chapter 4

The Six Myths Around Breast Cancer and How to Liberate Yourself from them and Enjoy a Life of Freedom and Happiness

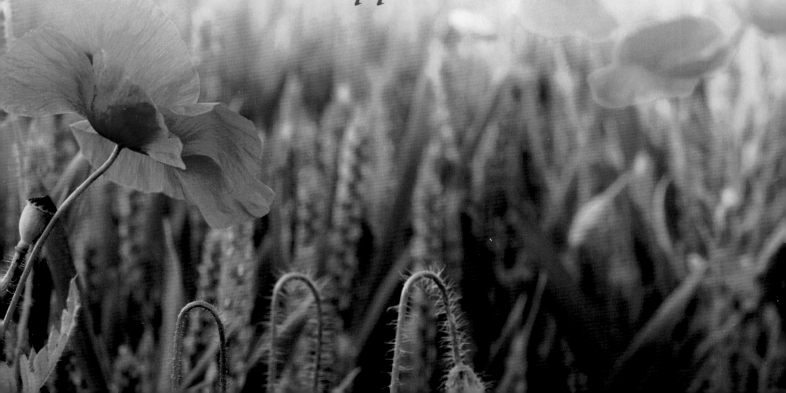

In this section, you will discover the six myths that keep people stuck and how you can free yourself and live fully. It is very important for you to know this, for otherwise you will continue to live in your current mindset or way of thinking yet expect a different result in terms of your health. This is the power of myths, for you have learned them from the time you were very young and have accepted them as the truth.

The benefits you will get from reading this chapter are:

- You will be making intelligent, conscious choices about when to see a doctor and when not to.

- You will give yourself more treatment options.

- You will discover how to get to the cause of your problem rather than just treating the symptoms.

- You will learn how to prevent illness in the first place.

- You will make a shift in how you view your health and live a magical life.

So What Are Myths and Why Are They Such a Huge Problem?

The Macquarie dictionary defines a myth as a collective belief system that is built up in response to the wishes of the group. In the context of this work, the group refers to doctors who have had the authority to influence patients or impose their beliefs upon them.

The body heals itself. The doctor picks up the bill.

(Mark Twain, Author)

The reason myths are such a huge problem is because they have become a part of your psyche, your unconscious mind. For example, when you were little, you would have learned that when you are sick, you see a doctor because only a doctor can heal you. This is a myth that Mark Twain's quote illustrates so succinctly. The fact is that the body is an amazing self-healing, self-restorative, and regenerative mechanism.

Myth Number 1:
There Is No Cure for Cancer

When most people hear this myth, they believe they are going to die. It arouses feelings of panic. It seems like a big deal. But it is just a popular myth – clearly, not everyone who has had cancer has died. If this were true, I would not be writing to you today.

In the book *The Cancer Conspiracy*, the writer, who is an employee of a large drug company, alleges that "the war on cancer is not being won – it's not even being fought. Why? There's no money in curing cancer – there's money in treating cancer." (Horn 2006: 104) I am rather perplexed about this sweeping statement, even about treatment, for breast surgeons often claim that nobody knows the cause of cancer and yet it has been found that "its incidence is less common among vegetarians."

You may be wondering what the treatment with medication is all about if no one knows the cause of cancer. Is it mere speculation based on anecdotal evidence? We are all too familiar with the placebo effect; and as Mark Twain's quote so succinctly puts it, the body would have healed itself anyway without the doctor.

Fact: From my own interactions with the medical fraternity, I am aware that not all doctors believe cancer is incurable. Most breast surgeons can assuage patients' fears of a recurrence of a malignant tumor in the same breast with the added caution that they be vigilant of its occurrence in the other breast or in the uterus or cervix as the patient may have a predisposition to cancer.

If you were such a patient, you would probably be making radical shifts in diet protocols, your lifestyle, and psycho-emotional health rather than living in the fear of manifesting a tumor in some other organ. There is a plethora of evidence that there is a cure for cancer. (See the DVD "Community of Commonsense Doctors," 2010.) This community consists of some forty doctors and cancer experts.

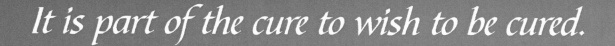

It is part of the cure to wish to be cured.

(Lucius Seneca, Roman Philosopher,
Statesman, Dramatist 4 BC– 65 AD)

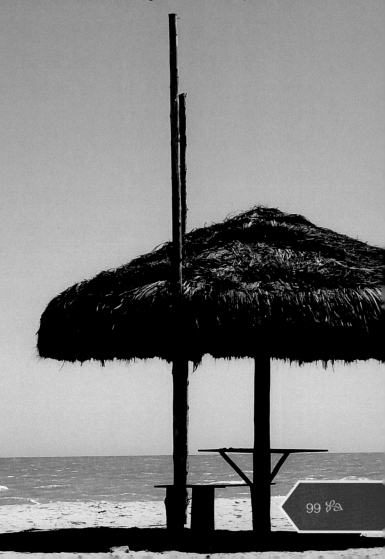

Much research has pointed to the fact that our mind plays an essential role in activating our innate self-recuperative potentialities. I like Louise Hay's (1987) redefinition of the word "incurable": it implies that the "particular condition cannot be cured by any outer means and that we must go within to find the cure." The answer lies within us.

In order to heal yourself, you will need to find the mental pattern of resentment or anger that has been turned inward (and not expressed). If you find this work too daunting, you may need the expertise of a therapist.

Dr. Norman Shealy (neurosurgeon) asserts that even when it is too late for prevention, the things that can assist in preventing cancer are recommended in its treatment – that is, treatment outside the traditional medical model of surgery, chemotherapy, radiotherapy, or drug therapy.

Myth Number 2:
Medications Such As Tomoxofin or Femara Can Treat Breast Cancer

What this myth implies is that if you were on these drugs, you would become healthy again; but this is not the case. The cure lies within YOU; drugs do not heal you. In fact, many studies have shown that tomoxofin can cause deafness.

Nothing is right or wrong, but thinking makes it so.

(Oscar Wilde, Writer)

Such medications are used as an adjunct to surgery, as a precautionary measure to prevent a recurrence. However, if one has been on certain doctor-prescribed medications for a prolonged period, these medications may have actually predisposed the person to having a weak immune system. In other words, taking certain medications may well be a part of the reason you got cancer in the first place, since certain drugs can suppress the immune system and cause weakness in the body.

Fact: Certain medications such as cytotoxic drugs do kill cancer cells, but these are not used for breast cancers but for other forms of cancers. It has been suggested that tomoxofin may be effective after ductal breast cancer (in situ) surgery, but there is no evidence that it can kill cancer cells.

In fact, as I mentioned above, it is dangerous to be on any form of medication for a prolonged period. There is a great deal of evidence that taking certain doctor-prescribed medications over a long time can predispose a person to having a weak immune system and hence be a contributory factor in the growth of malignant tumors in the breast.

Some American and European studies have shown that doctors regularly prescribe placebos (i.e., fake pills) to help their patients, claiming that doing something is better than doing nothing. Placebos are given on the assumption that patients believe they will work, and research does show that they sometimes do work. On the other hand, it has been proven that nutritional and dietary treatments have a great track record for helping cancer patients. (See the DVD "Community of Commonsense Doctors," 2010.)

The body has its own pharmacy – as we learn to silence the cognitive surface mind through meditation or other spiritual practices, the universal mind has the intelligence to heal the body naturally – to produce the ideal amounts of hormones and balance the body's chemistry.

We are plugged into a limitless, in exhaustible supply of boundless energy. Let it flow through you vibrantly, unimpeded, harmoniously, continually nourishing and rejuvenating your body. James Frampton (Energy Practitioner)

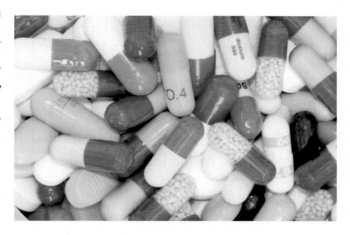

Myth 3:
Alternative/Complementary Medicine Is Quackery

What this myth means to most people is that complementary medicine is not safe; it is useless; it is dangerous; it does not work. It implies that if you do not see your doctor, you are wasting your time and money. What if you could dispel this myth by realizing you have the power to make your own choices?

Fact: There are thousands of real-life stories in which alternative healing modalities have been used to cure cancers naturally. These include psychological therapies (e.g., alternative healing modalities, psychotherapy), physical therapies (e.g., Ayurvedic medicine, nutritional therapy), spiritual healings, and many more.

In fact, in 2012 some medical boards in California called upon mainstream doctors to practice integrative medicine that supports what Hippocrates (the father of modern medicine) so succinctly spelled out in the quote on page 101.

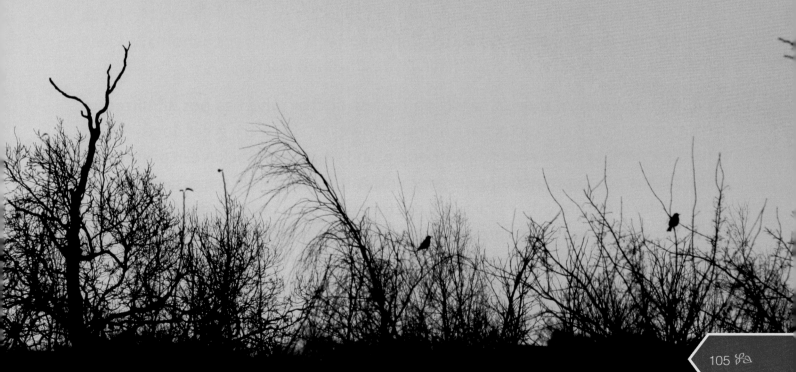

Health depends on a state of equilibrium among the various factors that govern the operation of the body and the mind; the equilibrium in turn is reached only when man lives in harmony with his external environment.

(Hippocrates, c.460–377 BC)

Myth Number 4:
Doctors Know Everythng; They Are Trained Medically

What this suggests is that only a doctor can have your best interests at heart and that you can reliably hand over your health to your doctor, that it is pointless seeing anyone else. However, the following facts will help you debunk this myth and take your life back into your own hands.

Fact 1: A doctor is just a person; "doctor" is just a job title. Doctors do not know everything. They are just people who have been put on a pedestal by society, as if their status comes next to God. We can all relate to Dr. Jekyll and Mr. Hyde and to many real-life doctors reported in the media worldwide who have killed patients due to medical errors. They were all trained doctors.

In my experience, there's hardly an honest doctor who has not admitted to having made an error. Doctors are human. However, there are great doctors who love their profession, love caring for people, and who do not believe in prescribing medications or recommending surgery unless it is absolutely necessary. On the other hand, there are other practicing doctors who have become doctors because their parents talked them into going to medical school because "the money is good and one gets to travel and have a great lifestyle." For many of these doctors, medicine may not have been their passion, and this raises doubts about their enthusiasm and competency.

Fact 2: It is now common knowledge that medical students are taught nutrition during only one or two lectures out of their six years of training – this is hardly scratching the surface.

We have heard only too often that we are what we eat. Hence, a sound knowledge of nutrition is very important in helping us make intelligent choices about food.

"…We live in an interactive reality where we change the world around us by changing what happens inside of us while we're watching - that is, our thoughts, feelings, and beliefs…. From the healing of disease, to the length of our lives, to the success of our careers and relationships, everything that we experience as 'life' is directly linked to what we believe."

(Gregg Braden – author, speaker)

Myth Number 5:
The Gene Theory: Cancers Run in the Family and Cannot Be Prevented

What this means for you is that if your mother had breast cancer, you are likely to get it too because it is in the genes. Nothing could be further from the truth. You can dispel this myth and live a fear-free life as evidenced by the following research:

Fact 1: One's genetic predisposition to any disease is less than 5 per cent, and even in these cases, the propensity can be totally alleviated by altering one's environment, lifestyle, and dietary patterns. (Dr. Bruce Lipton – DVD)

Some research shows that most of the patients within the 5 per cent genetic predisposition do not develop the disease. (Dr. Sangeeta Pati)

Fact 2: Research in the field of Energy Medicine suggests that if a person buys into this myth and gets cancer, it may well be because his or her thoughts and emotions are powerful. If you keep thinking along the lines of "My grandmother had breast cancer, my mother had it, and my aunt had it" and dwell in this negative energy, it is highly probable that you may well end up growing a malignant tumor yourself. You will find what you think about. Your thoughts are powerful, so it is vital to be aware of one's self-talk.

Live lightly and freely as a bird to promote radiant health, joy and longevity

(Dr Pargash Giorgi)

 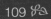

Myth Number 6:
Single Women Who Have Not Had Babies Get Breast Cancer

What this myth means to most women is that if they have had children, they are not likely to get breast cancer. But this is not necessarily true, for such cancers are as prevalent among women who have had babies as those who have not.

Fact: Superficially, this myth would make sense, for during your reproductive age, you go through significant hormonal changes each month. It is your body's way of preparing itself for "becoming a milk organism . . . shifting from a resting state to a prepared state to produce milk." (Dr. Alexander Splatt, radiologist, personal communication) However, this is just a myth. Women who have had children are just as likely to get breast cancer as nuns, single women, and married women who have not had babies.

Are you willing to release the above myths? If so, please repeat the following affirmation many times over a week. It might be a good idea to say this affirmation standing in front of a mirror:

I . . . (your name) hereby commit to enjoying a myth-free, healthy and vibrant life.

For more information please visit my website
newlifeafterbreastcancer.com
for a free one-on-one session on how to get your life back on track, during which I deliver the **transformational experience** that will set you *free*. And don't forget to pass this invaluable information on to your friends and family too.

Thank You!

You have seen it before and you will see it again, so have faith: what feels now like an impassable mountain, or a massive stumbling block, is in fact your stepping stone.

(Brian Vaszily)

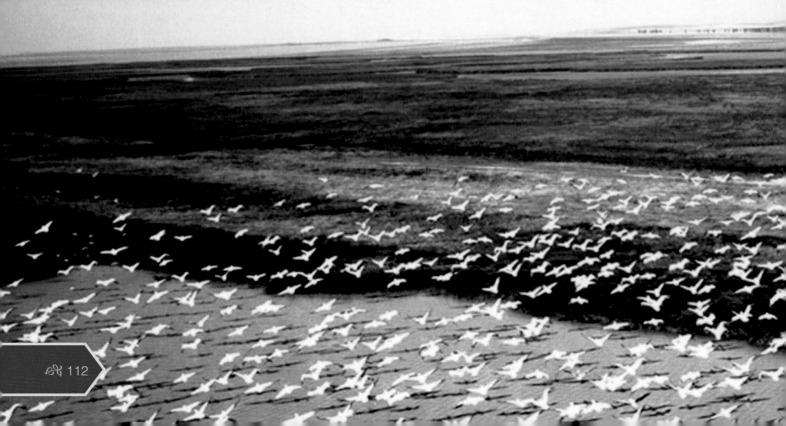

Once you unlearn what you have been conditioned to believe, the key to your unlimited power will be unlocked.

(Joshua Bloom, Founder of Quantum Energy Healing Center, NY)

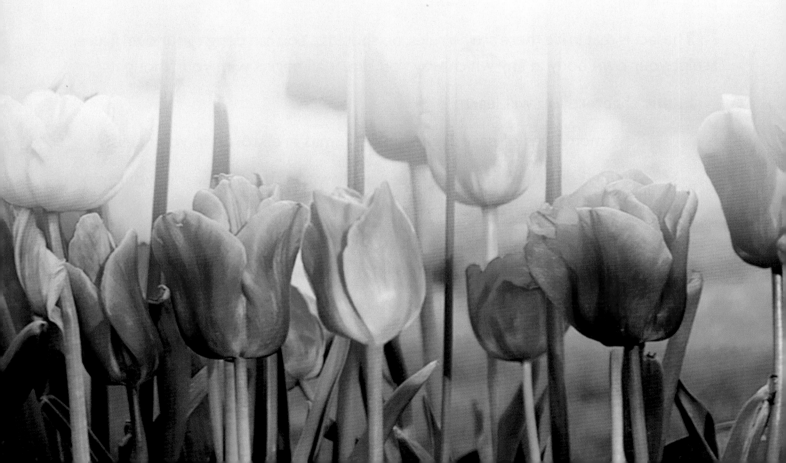

Chapter 5

How to Live a Cancer-Free, Happy Life Using the Power of Your Mind

Our thoughts create our reality. Our energy goes where our focus is; so if you choose to focus on your health and well-being and think such thoughts that feel right for you, that make you feel good, then you can't help but manifest happiness and vibrant health. Having a positive mental attitude is the key to your health and well-being. Your attitude consists of your thoughts, feelings, and actions.

We have all been programmed by the media and women's magazines as to how our bodies "should" look to be attractive and beautiful. We bought into these false conditionings. As Joshua Bloom's quote (page 109) points out, this is false programming.

The fact is that in life there are no rules, no shoulds. You can design your own figure, sculpt your own body in any which way you like. It all begins with your thoughts.

In this chapter, you will learn:

- how memories of past events and traumas are stored in your cells;

- cutting-edge tools and techniques on how to use the power of your mind to remove the negative charge around these memories;

- how to use cutting-edge tools and techniques to install new, positive, and life-enhancing thought patterns and reinvent yourself.

The subtle difference between thriving and surviving is solely based upon a memory resonating as a limiting belief or an imagination filled with infinite possibilities. Your brain and body don't know the difference. However, because the subconscious will always override the conscious [mind], the DNA that constructs the blueprint of who you are biologically and behaviorally resides in the light body of your chakras. Use your imagination and create your life through the power of intention!

(Dr. Darren Weissman)

Healing Modalities

There are many healing modalities that can assist you in healing your mind and emotions by resolving your psycho-emotional-spiritual issues, such as hypnotherapy, psychotherapy, breathing exercises, and many others.

The two common healing modalities in the field of Energy Healing are the Emotional Freedom Technique (EFT – also called Tapping) and Quantum Energy Transformation. The one I used on myself (the one I use continuously) is EFT, which involves using the power of intention to energetically remove the blocks or limiting beliefs and install new, empowering beliefs through affirmations or mantras.

Tapping is a quite revolutionary, energetic approach that is becoming rather trendy because it gets fast, lasting results. It is also gaining acceptance in medical communities due to the emergence of empirically based evidence, (Dawson Church, EFT Master, 2012). EFT goes to the root of your problem, making you emotionally resilient so that you can run *free* in life and explore new things.

To use the analogy of a guitar, tapping is like learning how to tune your guitar (your body) so that you can play beautiful music with your life because you will be in harmony with yourself and your Higher Self. Tapping will help you get in touch with your power and begin to compose the life of your dreams.

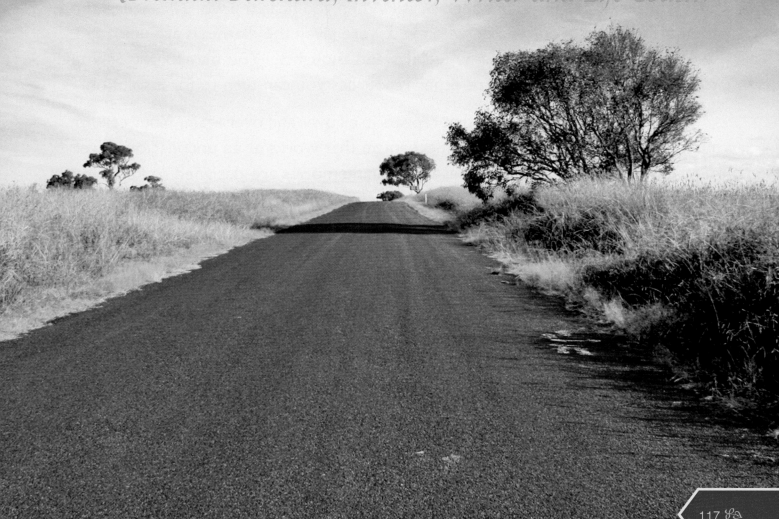

Life itself is energy, so if you have no energy, what does that say about your life?

(Brendan Burchard, Inventor, Writer and Life Coach)

Tapping helps you release the charge around your unproductive cellular memories that get activated or triggered by certain situations. It removes the roots of the tree, as it were. It helps you let go of the root cause of your problem so that you are no longer imprisoned by it. When you hear the word "cancer," the memories of how you reacted when you were given the diagnosis are uploaded, and you respond with the same feelings and thoughts. You may forget or you may be unaware that there are other resources you can turn to for a solution.

This is a destructive pattern that repeats itself over and over again. Your cellular memories are a form of survival mechanism that works at an unconscious level. (Dr. Sugar Singleton, 2011). These cellular memories are designed to keep you safe and to protect you, but all too often they can wreck your life. Your awareness of this pattern is the first step in your journey of healing; awareness helps you go beyond the symptom to the cause of your thought patterns, attitudes, behaviors, and feelings. Then you can move forward and live a thriving life.

You may say, "But if I have had surgery and radiotherapy, then I have gotten rid of these bad cells permanently." You are right. However, you would still want to address the root cause of why you got cancer in the first place so that you can live a fear-free life, free of the fear of tumors growing in other organs.

It is possible that you are identifying with certain thought patterns such as "I am not worthy/good enough" and that you are lacking self-acceptance at an unconscious level, at a cellular level. It is highly likely that you are not enjoying optimal self-esteem. But you can see your challenges as seeds to your greatness, as messages to tap into your highest potential.

Pure love, living and interacting in integrity, eliminates all dis-ease and ailments because it makes your cells super-happy. Love and disease can't co-exist, just as love and fear can't co-exist. Hence, falling in love with yourself is the first step to your permanent recovery – your first step to a happy, healthy, and joyful life.

The following six tools can assist you in your healing process now. As you use these tools, you will learn to love yourself, keep your heart open, allow your body to express its energy, enjoy an active, exuberant life, and transition into your life purpose.

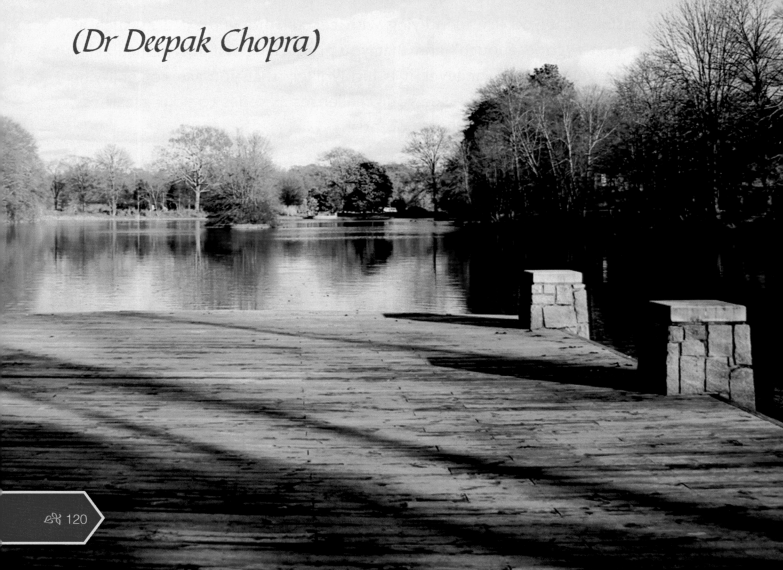

Fear and anxiety send up countless thoughts, but until you move the energy, attending to the thoughts will not bring lasting relief.

(Dr Deepak Chopra)

1. Tapping

It is completely natural to compare our breasts after surgery and feel self-conscious when we undress in the presence of our partners or lovers, but we can overcome this limitation. We can tap for creating self-love and acceptance and be okay with how we feel about our breasts. This will shift the energy.

It's best to stand in front of a mirror, nude if possible, when you do this tapping exercise. Focus on the part of your body (e.g., left breast) that you may not like to look at after the surgery. Now imagine it looking exactly as you want it to look. Imagine what it would feel like to have this "look" becoming real. Focus on what you do want continuously, as this will change your thought patterns. How do you want to feel when you look at your breasts? Feel those feelings now. Emotionalize the new you into being, totally accepting your body, no matter what.

Below is a diagram indicating the main tapping points.
For more details, please visit my website at

newlifeafterbreastcancer.com

to watch the EFT Video on *Secrets to Emotional Freedom After Breast Cancer*.
Please feel free to share this information with your friends and family.

Thank You!

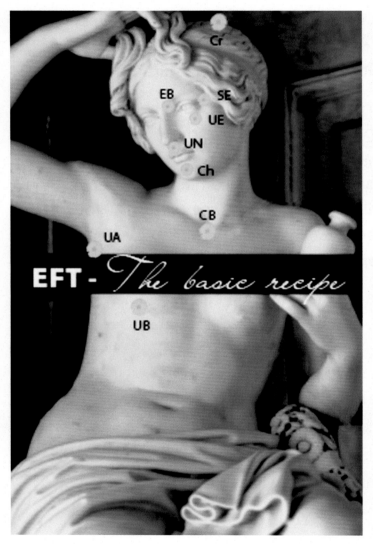

EFT - *The basic recipe*

On a scale of 1–10, rate the intensity of feelings that your breast evokes in you, and notice where in your body you feel them. Be specific about the feelings (e.g., whether you feel sadness or anxiety or fear) so that you can adapt to the following script:

Even though I don't like . . . (mention the specific part of the breast, for example, the way the left side of my left breast looks), I deeply and completely love and accept myself.

Even though I feel uncomfortable with the way my . . . (part of your breast) looks, I accept all my feelings, and I deeply and profoundly love, accept, and honor myself.

Even though I do not like certain aspects of . . . (part of your breast) and I can't help comparing and feeling a little sad, I deeply and profoundly love, accept, and forgive myself and everyone else who may have contributed to my feeling this way.

(Tap each of the tapping points listed below and say the accompanying affirmation.)

Eyebrow point: I don't like how (e.g., left or right... specific part of breast) looks.

Side of the eye: I really don't like . . . .

Under the eye: I wonder why I keep judging myself.

Under the nose: I feel sad/uncomfortable/anxious.

Under the mouth: All this sadness/anxiety/feelings of discomfort.

Collarbone: I do feel sad/anxious/scared.

Under the arm: Why am I stuck in this place?

Top of the head: All this sadness/fear/anxiety.

Eyebrow point: What if I released these feelings?

Side of the eye: These negative feelings toward my breast don't serve me.

Under the eye: They keep me stuck.

Under the nose: I picked up this pattern of negativity a long time ago

Under the mouth: When I did not know how to deal with these feelings.

Collarbone: But I'm much stronger and courageous now.

Under the arm: I can get clear and be open to loving and accepting my breasts

Top of the head: Exactly as they are, starting now.

Now take a deep breath and rate the intensity of your feelings again. It may have gone down or up. If it has gone up, continue with a few more rounds until it comes down to about 3 or 4. Then do a few more rounds starting with the eyebrow point, just saying, "I release and let go all remaining (specify your feeing)." Keep tapping until you get to 0.

Next, do a positive round of appreciation on what you like about your breasts. For instance, you could use phrases such as *I choose to love my breasts exactly as they are* or *I choose to appreciate the beauty of my breasts as they enhance my figure* or something to that effect. If it does not resonate with you, you will have to go back to tapping on your negative feelings over and over again until you can appreciate your breasts exactly as they are.

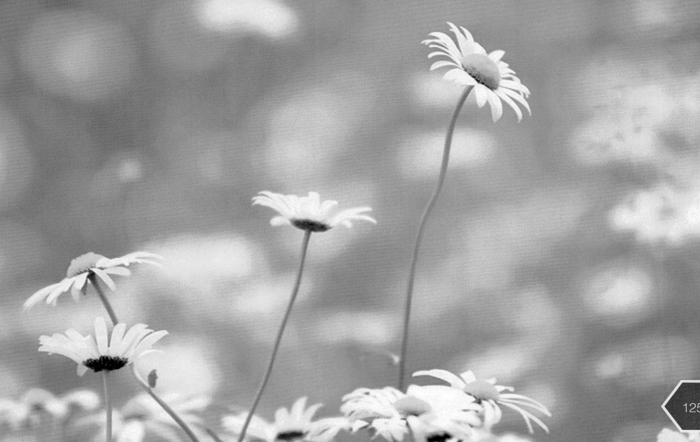

We act, behave, and feel according to what we consider our self-image to be, and we do not deviate from this pattern.

(Dr Maxwell Maltz, Cosmetic Surgeon, Author)

2. Writing/Journaling

It may also be helpful to write down your story such as I have in Chapter 1, as the process of writing is powerful in bringing up emotions. Then do as many rounds of tapping as you require to release all the feelings that get triggered by your memories – feelings such as sadness, anger, and so on. To check if you have released all the charge around those memories, reread your story and tap each time you feel any negative emotion. Do not resist any of your emotions, as resistance will only make them stronger.

3. Changing Your Inner Self-concept

It is essential to change your self-concept or self-image since doing so will shift your perception of who you are. Changing the perspective you want to live by can be miraculous. You must change those traits in you that no longer serve you because they are based on your external experiences. If you do not do this, you will be getting the same results as before. In other words, if you want to change your life, you must first want to change your self-concept. For example, if being a submissive/people-pleaser has not worked for you, learn to say no more, knowing that you need to change to the "new you" without any fear of rejection. If people love you, they will accept the change.

What Is the Inner Self-concept and How Does It Affect Your Life?

Before we discuss the inner self-concept, you first need to quickly remind yourself of who and what you are. Who or what is your authentic self?

As you already know on a deeper level, you are more than your body. You are more than your memories. You are more than your name, your job, and all your accomplishments. You are an eternal being, powerful beyond measure. Your thoughts, feelings, and states of consciousness are the cause of your external world/experiences. In fact, you are editing your Reality right now, and your editing facilities are based upon your beliefs, which have been programmed into you over a long period of time. Many of the things that you believe are not actually your own ideas. They are tribal, cultural, or religious conditionings (or subconscious imprints) that have no real relevance to you, your authentic self.

If all this conditioning were removed today, you would still exist and you would come to know who you really are. So it is a good idea to let go of the beliefs that do not work for you and replace them with those that inspire you to fully blossom as a woman.

According to a number of different sources from mystics to scientists, this physical world that we perceive is very similar to a hologram. We are living in a holographic universe that appears extremely real to us – but is in fact the consequence of things that we cannot see with our eyes. For more information about this holographic world, I suggest you read the book Holographic Universe by Michael Talbot.

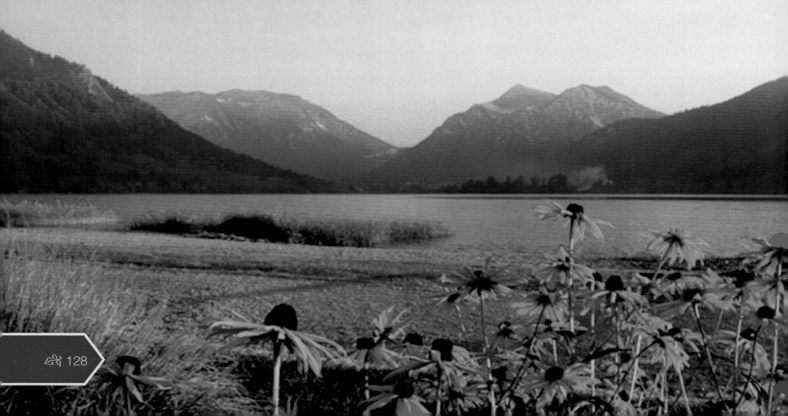

Whenever we change who we are for the sake of being accepted, we lose the infinite capacity and power to shine. The truth of who we all are is pure love. The increasing numbers of diagnoses of physical cancer is a direct link to how far away humanity has strayed from its connection to the spiritual truth of life itself.

(Dr. Darren Weissman)

How Is This Relevant to You and Your Life?

Right now, the combination of all your beliefs, experiences from the past, dreams, ideas, and every other kind of experience that you have ever had are all formed together in what I call your "Inner Self-Image or Self-Concept." Your Self-Concept is essentially a holographic plate that is currently manifesting the world you perceive around you right now.

As you change your beliefs, you change your life in dramatic ways. For example, if you buy into your cultural beliefs that women do not deserve to be prosperous, you will continue to perpetuate a scarcity mentality of not being enough or having enough. Even if you win a lottery, you will find ways of spending it all or losing it so that it is in alignment with your self-concept – of not being worthy.

On the other hand, if you now choose to let go of this erroneous belief and install a new belief such as "I am abundant" and assume the feelings of what it would be like to be abundant, you will attract abundance into your life. This is a universal law of nature.

People React to Your Self-Concept

All your behaviors have to be congruent with your self-concept, no matter what it is. Therefore, if you choose to love yourself, you love the way you look and you consider yourself to be very physically beautiful in your mind, heart, and gut; and others will treat you as beautiful. If you see yourself as confident, competent, successful, and self-assured, others will treat you in the same manner. The examples are endless.

The outside world is a reflection of what is going on inside of you. This applies to every single aspect of your life: your health, wealth, relationships, and your spiritual life. Down to the tiniest detail, you create the world you see based on this self-concept that is contained within your consciousness.

How Does Your Self-Concept Change?

You can change your self-concept by going into the secret world within yourself, by seeing your current self-concept (that no longer serves you), setting the intention of dissolving it, surrendering it to the eternal light that you are, and allowing your Higher Self to see a new self-image or your authentic self.

This can be done through many healing modalities such as meditation, listening to CDs that are specifically designed to aid you on this journey, or various other energy healing modalities. As with all things, it involves time and practice. Sometimes things can shift in the flash of an eye, but certain patterns may take a lot of work and the shifts you experience will be subtle.

Changing one's self-concept is not anything new – it has been suggested in various ways by various people throughout the ages. It is, however, something that most people simply fail to do. Because they fail to do it, their life doesn't change.

It is my desire that you recognize the power that you hold to sculpt your reality, the power you have to shift your self-concept and live the best life ever.

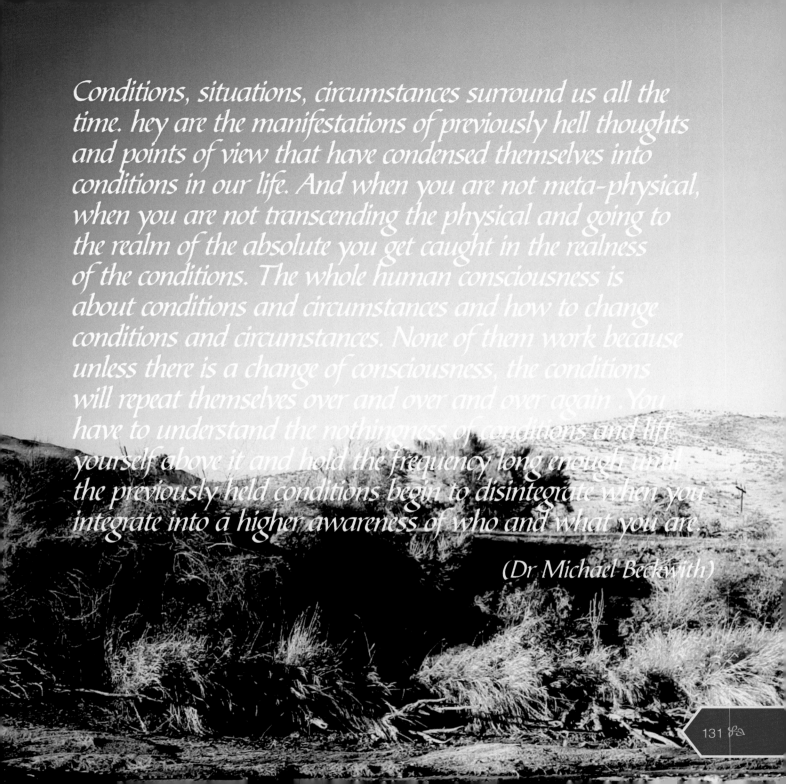

Conditions, situations, circumstances surround us all the time. hey are the manifestations of previously hell thoughts and points of view that have condensed themselves into conditions in our life. And when you are not meta-physical, when you are not transcending the physical and going to the realm of the absolute you get caught in the realness of the conditions. The whole human consciousness is about conditions and circumstances and how to change conditions and circumstances. None of them work because unless there is a change of consciousness, the conditions will repeat themselves over and over and over again . You have to understand the nothingness of conditions and lift yourself above it and hold the frequency long enough until the previously held conditions begin to disintegrate when you integrate into a higher awareness of who and what you are.

(Dr Michael Beckwith)

The Power of Surrender: The Secret to Health, Healing, and Happiness

It is essential for us to forgive and let go of what is bothering us for the following reasons:

- Most people who do not know about surrender and non-resistance struggle through life, making their problems worse despite the appearance that they are making things better.

- Once you learn to let go, your ability to self-heal multiplies.

- Letting go enables you to experience better relationships, less stress, more joy, and greater abundance.

So what is this all about?

All life has a natural self-healing and self-sustaining mechanism. No one tells a seed to grow or a tree to bear fruit or a chicken to catch a worm or a mouse to steal the cheese. These things happen because all life has a natural tendency to self-sustain.

The problem with our modern world and medical industry is we have become overly reliant on external forms of medicine and less reliant on our body's innate ability to heal. This has weakened our self-healing abilities, and we try to force things to happen rather than allowing them to happen of their own accord.

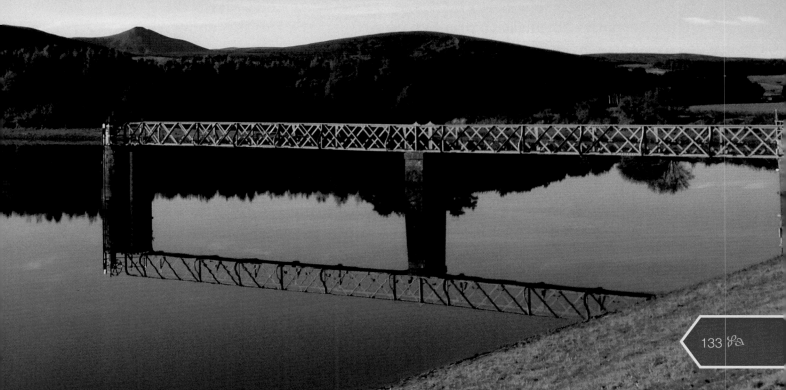

Your life is supposed to feel good to you, and you are meant to feel happiness in your life – and you are meant to satisfy your dreams….The more you practice good-feeling thoughts, the more you will allow unhindered cellular communication, and the more your physical body will thrive.

(Abraham Hicks)

Once you recognize and begin to appreciate the natural healing powers of your own body and soul, you will start to see little miracles happening in your life.

To begin with, you can try the following practices and see for yourself the profound effect.

Just let it go!

What most people do when they feel bad or are ill and have pain is to immediately try to force the feeling to go away. They stuff themselves with food to cover up feelings of depression, take an aspirin to get rid of a headache, or take some strong medicine to remove any symptoms of an illness. None of these things deal with the deeper cause of the symptoms and are merely a band-aid on a gaping wound that is still not healed and in most cases is getting worse.

The alternative to this is to practice non-resistance and surrender. Let go. As soon as you feel sad or sick, instead of medicating yourself to escape the pain, simply stop. Stop and BE with the pain. Allow it to be there. Allow yourself to feel the pain without any story. Don't try to figure out why it is there and how bad it is. Simply stop. Observe. Release the need to change it and surrender. Just watch it and let it be what it is. Breathe and allow. Imagine yourself surrendering to Source or whatever gives you an immense sense of gratitude for being alive. Tell yourself you are where you are and that it is okay to embrace this feeling. Bond with it until you come to a place of neutrality.

What you will notice as you stop resisting life and feelings is they tend to dissipate on their own in shorter spaces of time. They disappear and flow away like a river flows under a bridge. You will be amazed at your own self-healing and self-correction.

As you stop resisting life in general and surrender your life to a Higher Power, you will align with a much more powerful energy field than your own. As a result, your life will drastically improve.

Another powerful technique related to non-resistance and surrender is the process of letting go of the gratification we get from being "right" or repeatedly remembering past hurts and resentments.

When you have the choice to be right or to be kind, always pick kind. So many of your old thinking habits and their attendant excuses come out of a need to make yourself right and others wrong.

(Dr. Wayne Dyer)

So many people waste years of their lives in proving themselves right, trying to get even, and holding on to resentments. Holding on to resentments is like taking poison and expecting the other person to be ill. If you want a peaceful, meaningful life, it is essential to stop trying to be right and to let go of the past. You can profit from all the energy you have saved in negative emotions such as anger and resentment by directing that energy toward creating the life you want. All successful people know this secret. They are quick to let go of the past, quick to move on from a dispute and return to what is important to them.

If you do this you will have so much more energy and time that you'll be truly astounded. You can let arguments go without needing to prove your point. You can be free-flowing in life with grace and ease, fully focused on what brings you real joy, lasting peace, and a sense of happiness.

How to do this:

As a rule, do not engage in heated debates, arguments, or confrontation. Allow other people to be who they are while you focus your energy on the thoughts, words, and actions that align with your life's purpose.

Let go of the past. You wouldn't watch a bad movie over and over and over, would you? So stop recalling old memories in your mind. When negative thoughts come, welcome them and then let them pass like clouds in the sky. Move to thoughts of your heart's true desire and achieving what you want in life.

4. Oxy-breathing

Try this breathing technique recommended by Dr. Ellie Drake. Oxy-breathing stimulates the production of oxytocin, the female "love" hormone that is generally associated with love making and breast feeding. This type of breathing is especially good for women as it taps into our caring and nurturing "tend and befriend" natures. It is the perfect breathing technique for living a thriving life as a woman.

Whenever you feel like it's all too difficult or you are not good enough, you activate the fight/flight/freeze response. In other words, your ego gets activated while your soul becomes submissive. Oxy-breathing gets you out of a fight/flight/freeze state into a relaxed state.

The future belongs to those who believe in the beauty of their dreams.

(Eleanor Roosevelt – former First Lady of the U.S. and social activist)

Follow these steps and oxy-breathe daily, as often as you need to.

- Relax your shoulders.
- Relax your jaw and tongue.
- Make sure your feet are shoulder-width apart.
- Sit or stand, imagining a thread pulling your head toward the ceiling.
- Place your hand on/under your belly button and take a deep breath, ballooning your belly.
- Exhale with a long, pleasurable "haaaaa" sound/vibration (with a smile), or what Dr. Ellie Drake calls a "soulgasm." (With practice, you will soon find that when you place your hand on your throat, you will feel your throat vibrate as you exhale.)

The pleasurable "wind" sound tells your hypothalamus (the command centre of your brain) that all is well and you don't have go into a fight/flight mode. With practice, you will be tapping into the power in your belly to grow and evolve at your own pace. You will become fearless and free as you allow the power of love to flow through you in this relaxed state of tend and befriend.

In this spacious, relaxed state you may want to replace an unproductive belief such as "I'm not good enough" with a new, beneficial belief such as "I am enough" or "There is enough." You will feel good when you have such positive thoughts. Remember that a belief is just a thought you keep thinking habitually. So think thoughts that match your desires, keep thinking them until you believe them, and you will soon see the desired outcome.

Activate your potential. Real happiness does not lie in external accomplishments, or worldly things. Happiness, joy and ecstasy lie in the cultivation of your infinite and unique potential

(Dr Rev. Michael Beckworth)

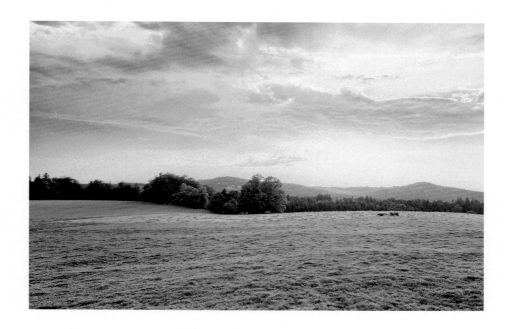

5. Singing

Singing (in an uninhibited manner with your mouth wide open!) releases emotional blocks related to your past. It vibrates the vocal cord muscles and releases unproductive cellular memories.

Below are the words of two healing songs that you can hum/sing to the tune of your choice (e.g., "Battle Hymn of the Republic"):

Song I

I am healed, whole and healthy

I am well, I am well

I am so blessed,

I feel wonderful

Thank you for this day (whatever evokes in you a deep sense of gratitude)

This healing day

There is only love

Love heals everything

I am ready to receive love, joy, and peace

I am ready to receive abundance and laughter

I love myself

I love my wonderful body

(Song written by Baerbel Froehlin – slightly adapted)

Song 2

I love myself so much

That I can love you so much

That you can love you so much

That you can start loving me

(Author unknown)

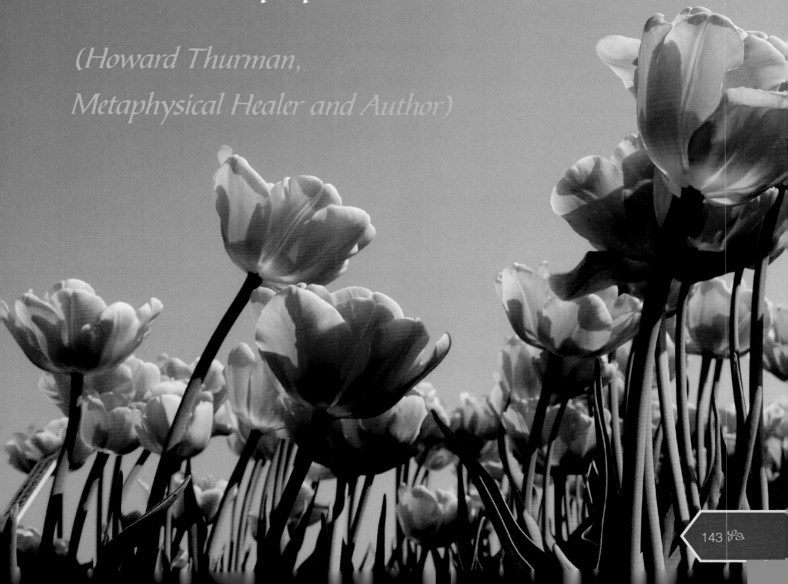

Don't ask what the world needs. Ask what makes you come alive, and go do it. Because what the world needs is people who have come alive.

(Howard Thurman,
Metaphysical Healer and Author)

6. Discovering Your Life's Purpose

Discover what you *really* want in life. As Howard Thurman's quote points out, it is key that you do what gives you the most joy. What matters most to you? Do you have a dream? Do you have a project you can unfold your life into? Most of us live a life that is driven by external circumstances, by our external programming that became set inside us as kids. We do not notice this until a life coach or some professional in the field of personal development points it out to us.

Do you have a reason for getting out of bed in the morning – your raison d'être? If you don't, it may be a good idea to reflect on what gives you the most joy. That will lead you to your life's purpose.

Some Practical Considerations

After you have taken the first step by working through the uncomfortable moments of indecisiveness to take action, do not expect too much too quickly. Healing and transformation can take time. Changing yourself is a full-time job, as we are never done. There is always room for improvement.

To learn more about my work, please visit my website at

newlifeafterbreastcancer.com

and claim your *free gift* valued at $585.

Be happy for this moment. This moment is your life.

(Omar Khayyam – Persian poet)

Don't cry because it's over, smile because it happened.

(Dr. Seuss – American writer, poet, cartoonist)

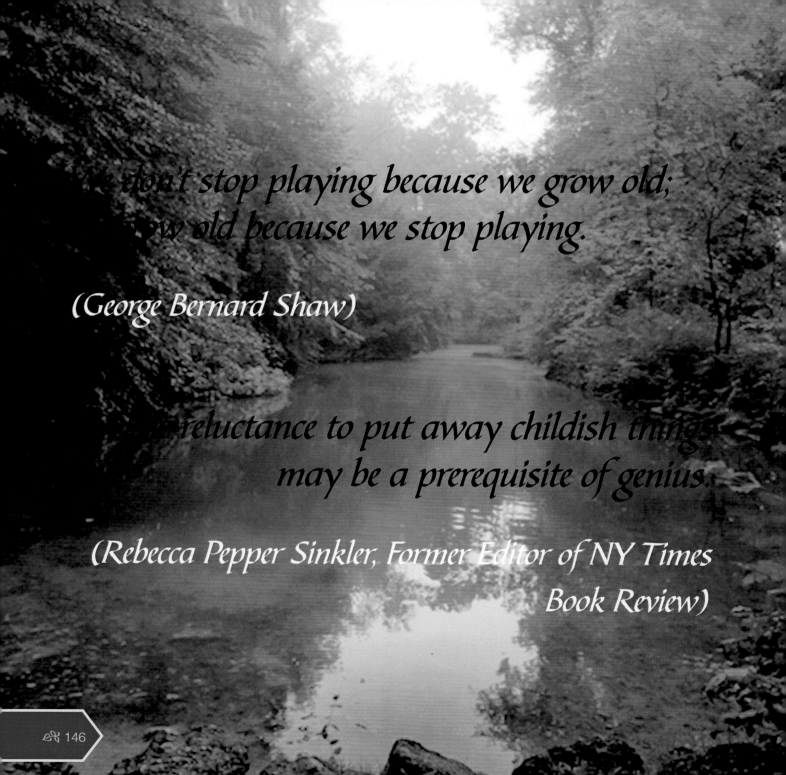

We don't stop playing because we grow old;
we grow old because we stop playing.

(George Bernard Shaw)

A reluctance to put away childish things
may be a prerequisite of genius.

(Rebecca Pepper Sinkler, Former Editor of NY Times
Book Review)

Chapter 6

Daily Rituals to Create Vibrant Health and Happiness

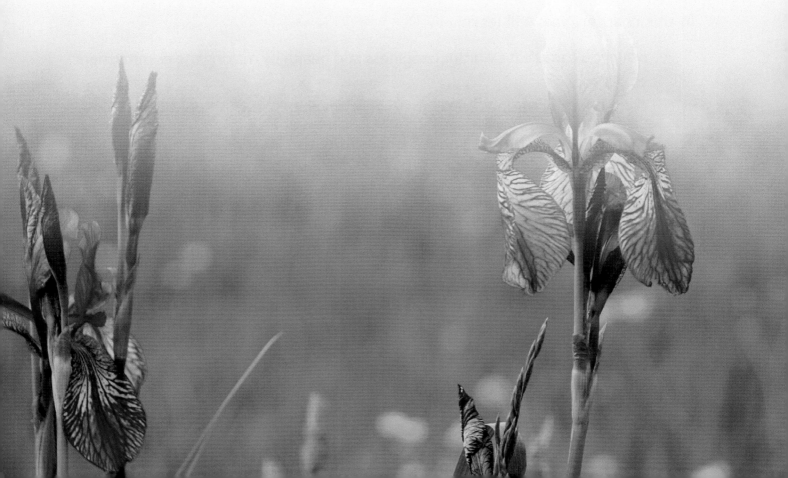

No matter where you are on your healing journey, it is absolutely necessary for you to let go of the past and to evolve out of the old mindset of "less than" and its thoughts like "I don't have enough energy" or "I don't have what it takes" into a new mindset of "I'm enough" and to see yourself as being fully cured and enjoying life to the fullest.

Remind yourself that you are now on a new path. You can change your life forever. You can shape your new abundant reality any which way you like. As the quotes above suggest, expand your playground and you will soon enjoy childlike energy and ignite your genius. Bring playfulness back into your life as you expand your comfort zone.

In this chapter, you will learn:

- how you can create vibrant happiness and health by making the commitment to do so;
- daily beauty routines for transformation that you can apply right away.

The ABCs of success in the sphere of creating the lifestyle that supports you are in reverse order –CBA:

C – Commit to creating a lifestyle that supports you in creating vibrant happiness and health.

B – Believe you *can* do it.

A – Take the necessary action steps and stay focused.

These three steps are crucial to your success. This commitment will transform your dreams into reality.

Love yourself first and everything else falls into line. You really have to love yourself to get anything done in this world.

(Lucille Ball – comedian, actress, and TV executive)

Something wonderful is always trying to happen through you, and it comes through your real identity. Meditation is the practice that clears the way for this conscious daily reconnection.

(Agape International - newsletter, 12 January 2020)

Your Choice of Daily Beauty Routines for Transformation

Immense satisfaction in life can be derived by taking pleasure in routines, so cultivate daily rituals/routines that are self-loving, ones in which you free yourself from all worldly pursuits and put yourself first, no matter what. You may want to set your alarm an hour earlier every morning. You absolutely need to make time for change.

Morning Regimes: Practice the first regime on the following list plus a few of the others that resonate with you, bring you joy, and saturate your tissues with oxygen.

- Drink a glass of water with some lemon juice upon waking. This will help flush out toxins. Aim to drink 2–3 litres of fluids per day between meals.
- Journal at least five things you appreciate in your life (e.g., your surroundings, your friends, and family). This is a powerful process of mental alignment with the laws of nature. Focus on what is going right in your world. I am sure you can write pages and pages of all the wonderful things for which you are grateful.

- Practice any type of meditation (detoxification of the mind) that resonates with you, preferably outdoors as the sun is rising. The golden light of the soft, morning sun is extremely healing and relaxing. It is safe to gaze at it while you are meditating. Begin meditating for ten minutes, gradually increasing it to thirty minutes. You may want to repeat a mantra such as I love and accept myself, no matter what.
- Tap to create self-love. (See Appendix B.)
- Sing/hum your favorite song.
- Dance a dance of your choice and/or indulge in your favorite exercise. If you are pressed for time, it might be a good idea to invest in a rebounder. It looks very similar to a mini-trampoline but is made with special piano springs. It exercises you at a cellular level and is sometimes referred to as a Cellerciser. It is great for you at any age and does wonders for lymphatic drainage. It also helps the immune system destroy pathogens, filter waste, and remove excess fluid and toxins. At the same time, it helps deliver vital nutrients and oxygen from the blood to the cells. Did you know that you have three to four times more lymph fluid in your body than blood?

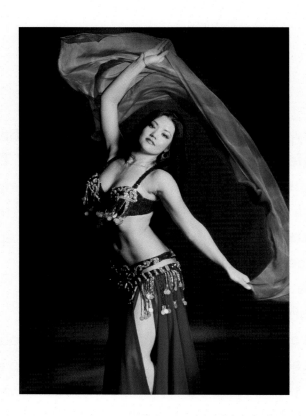

I dance as I rebound. You can even bounce holding dumbbells. Keep increasing the weight of the dumbbells as your strength increases. This is a super, time-efficient way to shape up and energize your life. It's a super-fast way of lifting your spirits too. Just get committed to your figure and *do it!*

For details on the Cellerciser, please visit the inventor's website at

www.cellercise.com

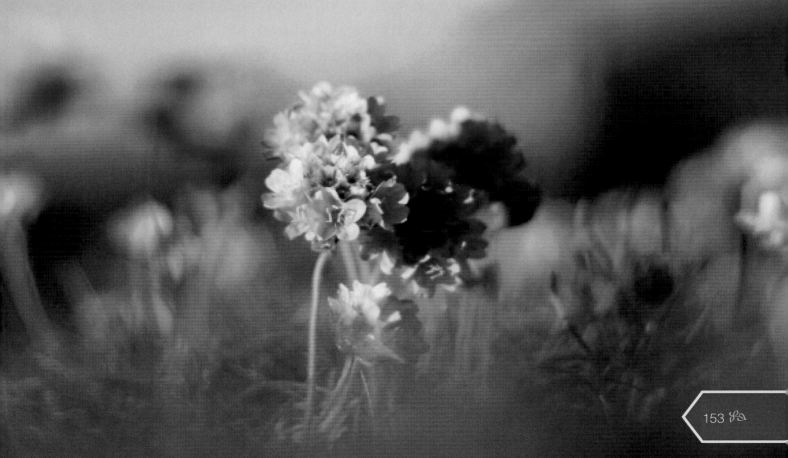

Once you become aware of who and what you are - pure consciousness - your body does not age because consciousness or awareness does not age. It is eternal and infinite. You can then choose your preferred biological age and re-create/sculpt your designer physique.

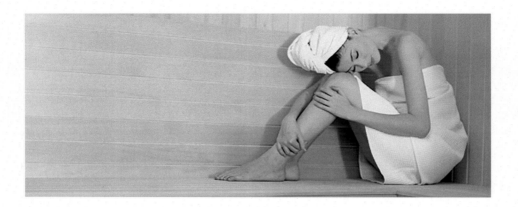

- Take an infrared sauna/hot bath for an instant sizzle. This is an *excellent* detox, especially if you have had radiotherapy and/or chemotherapy. The intense heat stimulates your immune system and strengthens your body. Cosmic-captivating inner radiance is just a by-product of it, the real beauty that comes from within. You will have glowing, gorgeous skin (your number-one beauty asset), and you will have the option to even wear the nude look. (I mean literally!) It guarantees an uplifting experience.

Evening Beauty Routines: Practice a few of the following that resonate with you.

- Repeat your meditation. (It would be great if you can do this at sunset, facing the sun.)

- Repeat your tapping for creating self-love. (See Appendix C.)

- Revisit your thoughts of the day and record fresh insights in your journal. For example, as you reflect on your day, ask yourself, "What did I learn today?" or "What could I have done differently?" You may find in hindsight that you might have done or said something differently. Our experiences change us daily.

• Read a chapter of a self-improvement book.

What sets successful people apart from the unsuccessful ones is that those who succeed make a habit of what they do not like to do. It is my desire that you will be committed to your success and be inspired to form some of these wonderful life-changing habits. They will help you liberate yourself and live your lofty dreams. They will propel you forward, powerfully and joyfully.

To learn more about our work, please visit our website:
newlifeafterbreastcancer.com

where you can register for our Live Event every week. Feel free to tell your friends and get them to join as well.

Thank You!

Because my lifestyle makes sense to me,
I'm immune to others' perplexed questioning,
and I'm never tempted to reverse my decision
to live as healthful an existence as I possibly can. My
rational determination to pursue optimal wellness
makes self-defeating choices unappealing.

(Dr Wayne Dyer)

Achievement seems to be connected with action....
Successful men and women keep moving. They make
mistakes, but they don't quit.

(Conrad Hilton)

157

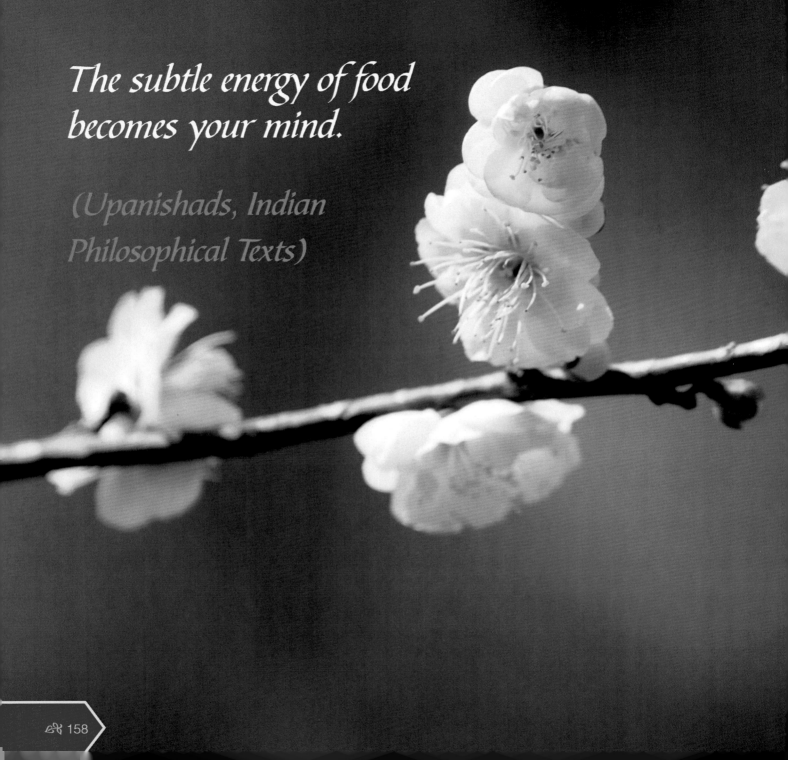

The subtle energy of food
becomes your mind.

*(Upanishads, Indian
Philosophical Texts)*

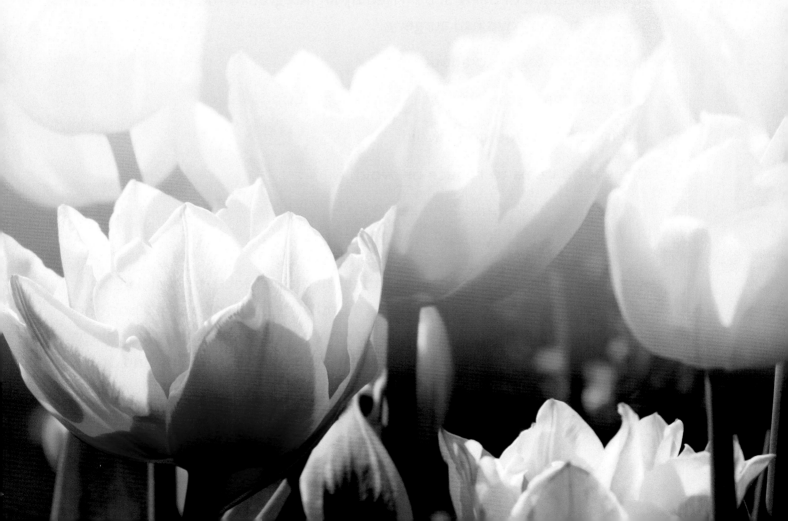

Chapter 7

Nutrition to Stay Cancer-Free

Nutrition is vital to rejuvenating one's mind, body, and spirit. As the quote (page 154) from the Upanishads suggests, the food you eat influences your thoughts. "It's easier to maintain a positive mental attitude if you're drinking wheat grass juice than soda pop. It's easier and you want to stack the odds in your favor." (Wolfe, D. Food Revolution Summit interview, May 3, 2012). You really are what you eat.

In this chapter, you will learn:

- the importance of being supervised by an integrative-medicine physician soon after you have had surgery;

- four key strategies to adopt;

- ten food items you must include in your diet;

- ten food items you must avoid;

- three food items to reduce or avoid.

Find a Well-known Integrative-Medicine Physician

It is very important to see an integrative-medicine doctor/physician who practices nutrition medicine for at least a few months, or until you are in a position to self-manage. This is because he or she will have you take the necessary pathology tests to see what is going on in your body in regard to minerals, vitamins, and other micro-nutrients. Until then, you may want to begin with the following action steps to ensure that you follow a balanced diet that will boost your immune system.

The food choices you make have an infinite power of restoring and regenerating your health, both internally and externally. You can choose to make the right food choices. For example, you can gradually replace a food program that is dominated by animal protein with one that consists of these three parts:

- one third protein (either animal and/or plant-based);

- one third sweet fruit (e.g., berries, cherries, apples);

- one third fatty food (e.g., avocados, seeds and nuts, and their oils).

The above food combination has tremendous benefits. You will enjoy abundant energy and stay at a higher frequency vibrationally. When you eat the right foods, you will also perform better, look great, and feel more beautiful.

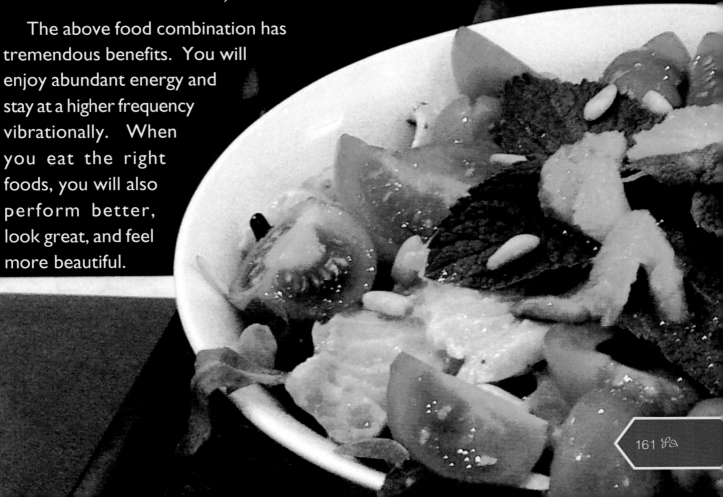

Four Key Strategies

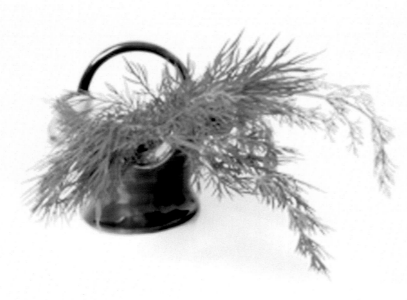

According to the world's leading experts on nutrition, such as David Wolfe and Gabriel Cousens, nutrition is as much about what you take out of your body as what you put in. As bad calcium is the cause of most diseases, it is key to adopt the following four strategies advocated by David Wolfe (2010). These strategies have worked for me and thousands of others.

1. Dissolve bad calcium through the use of bad calcium dissolvers such as citric acid, lemon juice, MSM crystals, and Celtic Sea Salt.

2. Incorporate herbal immune boosters (e.g., aged garlic extract, cloves).

3. Take cell-rejuvenating supplements and foods (e.g., enzymes, probiotics, Vitamin C).

4. Do deep-tissue bodywork and yoga, which will further break up calcification in your body. It is also a good idea to use an infrared sauna

if you have access to one, as it will help your skin detoxify and move lymphatic stagnation.

Ten Items You Must Include in Your Diet If You Are Serious About Your Health and Harnessing the Power of Your Innate Immune System

1. Drink 2–3 litres of fluids per day (e.g., vegetable juices, spring water, herbal teas, especially green tea). These will help your liver detoxify as well as provide your body with the right nutrients.

2. Cruciferous vegetables (e.g., kale, cabbage, broccoli) – preferably eaten raw as they are high-frequency energy foods and they are rich in antioxidants. They also help you detoxify the bad hormones from your body. They have powerful anti-cancer properties.

3. Seeds and nuts (sunflower seeds, chia seeds, Brazil nuts, macadamia nuts) – these will provide your body with the right minerals

4. Superfoods such as goji berries, raw cacao, noni, açai, spirulina, and chlorella

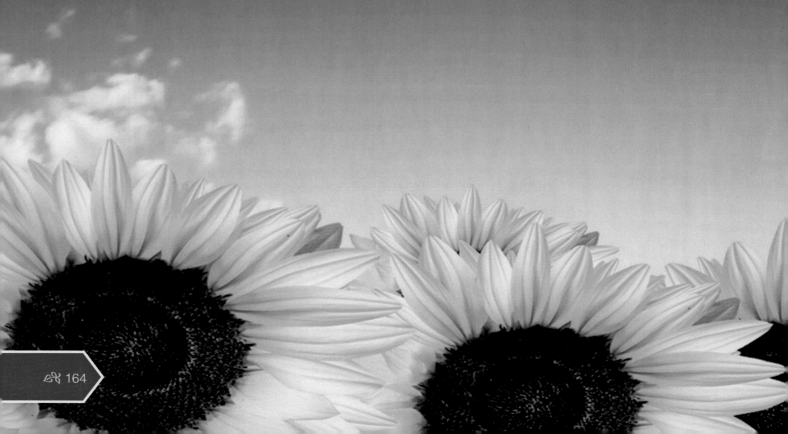

Let medicine be thy food. Let food by thy medicine.

(Hippocrates)

5. Mushrooms and mushroom extracts – a great source of protein with no calories

6. Avocados – they contain a great source of Omega-6

7. Aloe vera – it helps correct intestinal tract inflammation and aids absorption

8. Fish/krill/sea algae oil – great sources of Omega-3

9. Curcumin/turmeric extract and grapefruit seed extract – proven to fight tumors

10. Probiotics (e.g., sauerkraut or seed cheeses) – for a healthy gut terrain

These food items boost your immune system, your first line of defence. They are cancer-fighting foods.

Ten Items To Avoid (That Cancer Cells Love) To Restore and Regenerate Your Health

1. All sugar (as it feeds candida) apart from clear stevia or clear agave. It's easy to live sugar-free.

2. Gradually eliminate all dairy, cereal, and processed food, as they cause acidity and inflammation. Cancer cells thrive in an acidic environment.

3. All conventional meat and animal products because of their inflammatory component

4. All fast foods, as they contain toxic preservatives and are not nutritious

5. All non-organic fruits and vegetables, as they contain pesticides and other harmful chemicals

6. Eliminate all foods that contain aspartame (a food additive that is added to breath mints, hot chocolate, frozen foods, and other food items).

7. Processed table salt, as it contains a semi-toxic halogen mineral (Use Celtic Sea Salt instead.)

8. Foods with hydrogenated oils (e.g., French fries, fish fingers, crackers), since they contain trans-fatty acids that can disrupt your brain chemistry and cause much damage to your overall health.

9. All soft drinks, since they are loaded with sugar. Diet coke contains both aspartame and caffeine, which is a deadly combination.

10.   Tap water, as it contains more than 700 organic chemicals that may cause cancer.

Three Items To Reduce or Avoid If Possible

1. Alcohol, as it has a toxic effect on the body and can cause nutrient deficiencies

2. Cooked food – You lose a lot of nutrients and enzymes by cooking the food. If you must eat cooked food, have a salad with it, as the enzymes in the raw vegetables will catalyze the cooked food.

3. Meat and all animal products because of their inflammatory component

The above is just a summary of a good, anti-cancer diet protocol. The full version is beyond the scope of this book. Please refer to David Wolfe's book *The Longevity Now Program: The Most Precise and Comprehensive System for Achieving Total Health and Vital Longevity* for details and other cutting-edge information on nutrition.

Some Basic Recipes That You Can Prepare in Less Than Ten Minutes

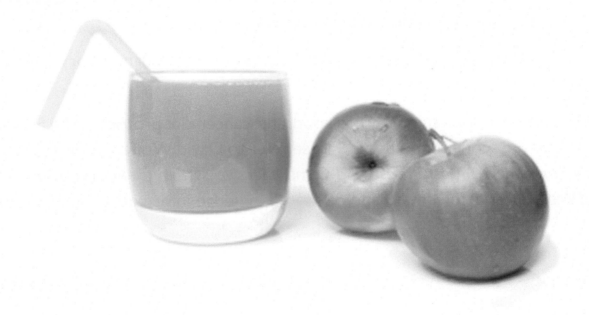

Breakfast

I cup blueberries (fresh or frozen)

I tablespoon of your favourite protein powder

1/2 teaspoon ginkgo biloba powder (boosts your brain)

1/6 teaspoon turmeric extract

I tablespoon of sunflower seeds or soaked chia seeds

An egg yolk (organic)

2 tablespoons organic coconut oil

I tablespoon flaxseed oil

Organic almond milk or rice milk

Blend for about 30 seconds

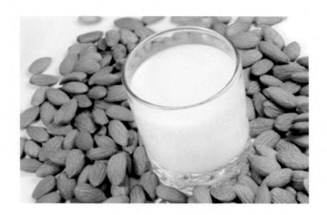

Lunch

A rainbow-coloured salad

A few strips of yellow and/or red capsicum

One or two radishes

Wild rocket and/or watercress

A dried fig – chopped

A few leaves of mint

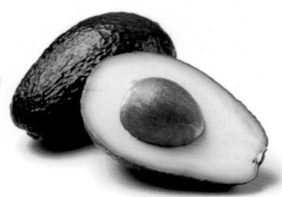

Capers

1/2 an avocado

A slice of yellow onion

Some seaweed (e.g. dulce)

Oil of your choice for a salad dressing (e.g. olive or coconut)

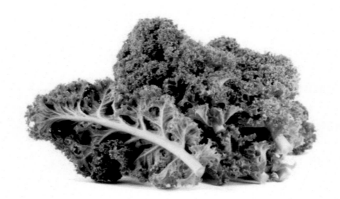

Blended Vegetables

Broccoli or cauliflower florets or Brussels sprouts

1 cup kale

1/2 cup cashews (rinsed) or almonds that have been soaked overnight

One avocado

A slice of yellow onion

1 or 2 pips of garlic

1/2 a teasppon of fresh ginger or turmeric

A pinch of cayenne pepper

Almond milk

Blend and add some coconut oil or olive oil just before eating. Or you may want to lightly steam your vegetables (e.g., okra, sweet potato, peas, pumpkin) and add your favorite oil, and have some smoked salmon or sardines with them.

Dinner
An elixir

Juice of one coconut

Meat of one coconut

Gel of a fresh aloe leaf

1/2 teaspoon marine phytoplankton

Fish oil or sea algae oil

2 tablespoons coconut oil

Blend for about 30 seconds

Beetroot, carrot, and apple salad

Grate a small beetroot

Grate a small carrot

Grate a Granny Smith apple

Garnish with some fresh coriander or mint

Sunflower seeds

Lemon juice/olive oil/coconut oil for the dressing

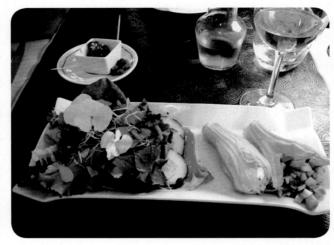

Snack yourself youthful on macadamia nuts, pumpkin seeds, sunflower seeds, berries, cherries, and wild strawberries.

Avoid eating anything four hours prior to going to bed so that you can sleep well and wake up well-rested and refreshed. You may want to have a hot chocolate before going to bed if you feel like having a warm drink.

A mind that is stretched by a new experience can never go back to its old dimensions.

(Oliver Wendell Holmes, Physician, Poet and Jurist)

To learn more about my work, please visit my website at

newlifeafterbreastcancer.com

where you can register to claim your *free gift* valued at $585. Feel free to tell your friends and family about it too so they can claim their gift as well.

Thank You!

REFERENCES

Allen, J. (2009) *As a Man Thinketh*. London: Penguin Group.

Beckwith, M., (2000) 40 Day Mind Fast, Soul Feast. A Guide To Soul Awakening. Agape Media International. LLC.

Beckwith, M., (2009) Spiritual Liberation: Fulfilling Your Soul's Potential. U.S., Simon and Schuster.

Carrington, P. (2008) Discover the Power of Meridian Tapping. USA: Try It Productions.

Chopra, D. (2008) *Ageless Body, Timeless Mind*. London: Random House.

Chopra, D. (2010) *Reinventing The Body, Resurrecting The Soul*. London: Random House.

Chopra., D. & Menas, K., (2017) You Are The Universe: Your Cosmic Self and Why It Matters. Penguin Books.

Drake, E. (2006) *It's Easier Done Than Said*. GA, USA: BraveHeart Productions.

Dyer, W. (2009) *Excuses Begone!* California: Hay House.

Dyer, W. (2010) *The Power of Intention*. California: Hay House.

Giorgi, P. (2001) *The Origins of Violence by Cultural Evolution*. Brisbane: Minerva E & S.

Hasset, J. (1984) *Psychology in Perspective*. New York: Harper & Row.

Hay, L. (1987) *You Can Heal Yourself.* Sydney: Hay House.

Holmes, Ernest. This Thing Called Life. 1948 Dodd, Mead & Co.

Horn, S. (2006) *POP!* New York: Penguin.

Look, C. (2008) *Attracting Abundance with EFT.* USA: Crown Media.

Look, C. (2012) *Emotional Freedom Technique in "Everything is Energy"
Teleseminar Series.* USA.

McKenna, P. (2009) *Control Stress.* London: Bantam Press.

Meares, A. (1981) *Relief Without Drugs.* Melbourne: Fontana.

Nuland, S. (1992) *Medicine: The Art of Healing.* New York City: Hugh Lauter.

Poole, W. (1993) *The Heart of Healing.* Atlanta: Turner Publishing.

Shealy, N. (1996) *Alternative Medicine.* Virginia: Element Books.

Singleton, S. (2011) *Cellular Memory in BraveHeart Women.* Vol. 1, Los Angeles:
BraveHeart Women Publishing.

Wilkes, R. and Vartuli, C. (2011) *Transform Your Emotions with Energy Tapping.*
USA: Ebook.

Wolfe, D. (2009) *Eating for Beauty.* Berkeley, California: North Atlantic Books.

Wolfe, D. (2010) *The Longevity Now Program.* USA: David Wolfe.

Wolfe, D. (2012) The Sunfood Diet Success System. Berkeley, California: North
Atlantic Books.

Wolfe, D. and Good, N. (2008) *Amazing Grace.* California: North Atlantic Books.

Wolfe, D. and Holdstock, S. (2005) *Naked Chocolate.* California:
North Atlantic Books.

AUDIOS

Beckwith, M., (2019) Prosperity, Plentitude & Infinite Possibilities.

Beckwith, M., (2012) Transcendence Expanded, Agape Media Hay House.

Church, D. (2012) *Scientific and Psychological Research Providing Evidence-Based Proof
that EFT and Tapping Work.* Interview with Gene Montrastelli on tappingqanda.com.

Massaro, Bentinho. Trinfinity Academy, 2016.

Yates, B. and Jones, S. (2010) *Confidence Beyond Belief.*

Yates, B. and McIntyre, D. (2010) *Beauty Beyond Belief.*

BestDayEver.com – David Wolfe interviewing Dr. Sangeeta Pati (January 2012) on breast cancer at the Women's Wellness Conference, Costa Mesa, California..

DVDS

Beckwith, M., (2000) Life Visioning Kit: A Step by Step Process for Realizing Your Highest Potential, Amazon.

"Cancer Is Curable *Now*" – Directors Cut by Community of Commonsense Doctors: maxAwareness.com 2010.

Craig, G. EFT Foundational Library; EFT Intermediate Library; EFT Honors Library.

Dyer, W. *There Is a Spiritual Solution to Every Problem.*

Lipton, B. *The New Biology—Where Mind and Matter Meet.* Distributed by Spirit 2000 Inc., 2001.

Lipton, B. *Nature, Nurture and the Power of Love – The Biology of Conscious Parenting.* Distributed by Spirit 2000 Inc., 2002.

Lipton, B. *As Above, So Below – An Introduction to Fractal Evolution.* Distributed by Spirit 2000 Inc., 2005.

Lipton, B. and Rob, W. *The Biology of Perception & the Psychology of Change of the Series Piecing it All Together.* Distributed by Spirit 2000 Inc., 2001.

LECTURE NOTES

Bloom, J. (2012) *Quantum Energy Transformation.*

Giorgi, P. (2000) *Functional Neuroanatomy.*

WEBSITES

www.agapelive.com

www.davidwolfe.com

www.thebestdayever.com

www.CancerIsCurableNow.tv

www.youtube.com/bradyates

www.thrivingnow.com

www.braveheartwomen.com

APPENDIX A
TAPPING SCRIPT FOR RELEASING YOUR FEARS AROUND HEALTH-RELATED ISSUES

Step 1: Take three deep breaths.

Step 2: Tune in to your feelings/frustrations – be as specific as possible for best results – Where in your body do you feel these feelings?

Step 3: Rate the intensity of your feelings on a scale of 1–10 and begin the tapping. Feel free to change the wording to suit your situation.

Even though I have all these fears, I deeply and completely love and accept myself.

Even though I am afraid to release these fears,

I deeply and profoundly love, accept, and honor myself.

Even though I have all these fears and frustrations, they seem so real, I choose to be calm and peaceful and I choose to love and accept myself anyway and anyone else who may have contributed to these fears and frustrations.

EB: I have so many fears.

SE: I have all these crazy fears and frustrations. (Be specific; for example, where in your body?)

UE: I have fears of a relapse.

UN: I don't want dis-ease in my body again.

UM: But I have all these fears.

CB: This resistance to taking charge of my health is all about fears.

UA: I remember the pain I went through.

TH: No wonder I don't want to release my fears.

EB: What if I could release some of my fears?

SE: I did survive and feel strong now.

UE: I can allow myself to process my experiences and move forward.

UN: I thank my body for all the amazing healings it does both consciously and unconsciously.

UM: I give myself permission to release all my fears and frustrations.

CB: I give my body permission to release all my fears and frustrations.

UA: I can choose to feel safe and the best ever even during this recovery process.

TH: I am grateful for my improving health.

EB: I choose to let go of all my fears.

SE: I choose to feel calm, relaxed, and confident.

UE: I choose to change my way of looking at my life.

UN: I allow myself to feel strong and confident.

UM: I allow myself to feel the best ever all the time.

CB: I allow myself to see myself and others with love.

UA: I am willing to see new possibilities.

TH: I choose to have my life go extraordinarily well all the time.

Take a deep breath. On a scale of 1-10, notice how intense your feelings are now. Tapping is a form of soothing yourself. It makes you less scared and more empowered. If you did not feel any shift in intensity, keep tapping a few more rounds until you feel it's easier to cope with your feelings and thoughts.

APPENDIX B
TAPPING FOR SELF-LOVE (MORNING RITUAL)

EB: I choose to love myself today.

SE: I choose to love, accept, and respect myself.

UE: I choose to love, accept, and forgive myself

UN: And anyone else I meet today.

UM: I may doubt that I am lovable.

CB: And I choose to release those doubts.

UA: They are just false programming.

TH: So I choose to clear them, for they don't serve me or anyone else.

EB: Clearing them at a cellular level.

SE: Clearing all thoughts of fear that get in the way.

UE: Clearing them all the way back to my past.

UN: I am worthy of loving myself and feeling great.

UM: I choose to flow through the day with an open mind.

CB: And I choose to love, honor, and accept myself today.

UA: I am willing to feel the best ever all day long

TH: In body, mind, and spirit.

APPENDIX C
TAPPING FOR SELF-LOVE (EVENING RITUAL)

SH: Even though things may not have gone perfectly well today, I choose to love and accept myself.

Even though (mention what did not go well), I choose to deeply and completely love and accept myself.

Even though (mention what did not go well) and I could have done it differently, I accept all my feelings, and I choose to love, accept, and forgive myself and anyone else who may have contributed to my feeling "less than."

EB: I choose to love and accept myself.

SE: I choose to really love and accept myself.

UE: And I choose to let go of all that did not go well.

UN: I did the best I could, given the circumstances.

UM: So I choose to love, accept, and forgive myself.

CB: Clearing any blocks that get in the way.

UA: Clearing them at a cellular level.

TH: And I choose to release the day as I peacefully drift off to sleep, knowing that tomorrow will take care of itself.

APPENDIX D

TAPPING FOR FORGIVING SELF

Even though I have made mistakes in the past, and I feel so guilty about what I have done, I love and accept myself anyway.

Even though I have been punishing myself for feeling guilty, I choose to release the guilt now.

Even though the guilt is trapped in my cells, I choose to love, accept, and forgive myself, and forgive myself no matter what.

EB: I have made mistakes in the past, and I have this overwhelming feeling of guilt in my body.

SE: I feel very guilty about my past mistakes.

UE: And I blame myself for those mistakes.

UN: I don't deserve to forgive myself.

UM: I'm not ready to forgive myself yet.

CB: I feel so guilty for all my mistakes.

UA: All this overwhelming guilt for things said or not said.

TH: I don't feel ready to let go of this guilt.

EB: What if I could release some of my guilt

SE: Just as I would forgive others for their wrong doings?

UE: I deserve to be free of my trapped emotions.

UN: I choose to release the guilt around what I did or said.

UM: I can allow myself to let go of the resistance to forgive myself.

CB: I have held on to this guilt for too long.

UA: I have been punishing myself for years and it is time to let go.

TH: I so appreciate this clarity.

EB: I'm so done with punishing myself.

SE: I am grateful for releasing this emotional poison of guilt.

UE: No wonder I had health problems.

UN: I deserve to forgive myself and move on.

UM: I can feel myself releasing the guilt and feeling lighter.

CB: It feels really good to let go of this burden of guilt.

UA: I appreciate my radiant health.

TH: I am grateful for this clarity in my life.

Printed in the United States
by Baker & Taylor Publisher Services